U.S. Department of Justice
Office of Justice Programs
National Institute of Justice

Guide for the Selection of Personal Protective Equipment for Emergency First Responders (Percutaneous Protection—Apparel)

NIJ Guide 102–00, Volume IIc

Dr. Alim A. Fatah[1]
John A. Barrett[2]
Richard D. Arcilesi, Jr.[2]
Charlotte H. Lattin[2]
Charles G. Janney[2]
Edward A. Blackman[2]

Coordination by:
Office of Law Enforcement Standards
National Institute of Standards and Technology
Gaithersburg, MD 20899–8102

Prepared for:
National Institute of Justice
Office of Science and Technology
Washington, DC 20531

November 2002

This document was prepared under CBIAC contract number SPO–900–94–D–0002 and Interagency Agreement M92361 between NIST and the Department of Defense Technical Information Center (DTIC).

NCJ 191521

---

[1] National Institute of Standards and Technology, Office of Law Enforcement Standards.
[2] Battelle Memorial Institute.

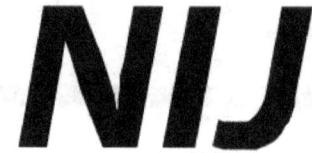

National Institute of Justice

Sarah V. Hart
Director

This guide was prepared for the National Institute of Justice, U.S. Department of Justice, by the Office of Law Enforcement Standards of the National Institute of Standards and Technology under Interagency Agreement 94–IJ–R–004, Project No. 99–060–CBW. It was also prepared under CBIAC contract No. SPO–900–94–D–0002 and Interagency Agreement M92361 between NIST and the Department of Defense Technical Information Center (DTIC).

The authors wish to thank Ms. Kathleen Higgins of the National Institute of Standards and Technology, Mr. Bill Haskell of SBCCOM, Ms. Priscilla S. Golden of General Physics, LTC Don Buley of the Joint Program Office of Biological Defense, Ms. Nicole Trudel of Camber Corporation, Dr. Stephen Morse of Centers for Disease Control, and Mr. Todd Brethauer of the Technical Support Working Group for their significant contributions to this effort. We would also like to acknowledge the Interagency Board for Equipment Standardization and Interoperability, which consists of Government and first responder representatives.

FOREWORD

NIJ is the research, development, and evaluation agency of the U.S. Department of Justice and is solely dedicated to researching crime control and justice issues. NIJ provides objective, independent, nonpartisan, evidence-based knowledge and tools to meet the challenges of crime and justice, particularly at the State and local levels.

The NIJ Director is appointed by the President and confirmed by the Senate. The Director establishes the Institute's objectives and is guided by the priorities of the Office of Justice Programs, the U.S. Department of Justice, and the needs of the field. The Institute actively solicits the views of criminal justice and other professionals and researchers to inform its search for the knowledge and tools to guide policy and practice.

In partnership with others, NIJ's mission is to prevent and reduce crime, improve law enforcement and the administration of justice, and promote public safety. By applying the disciplines of the social and physical sciences, NIJ:

- Researches the nature and impact of crime and delinquency.
- Develops applied technologies, standards, and tools for criminal justice practitioners.
- Evaluates existing programs and responses to crime.
- Tests innovative concepts and program models in the field.
- Assists policymakers, program partners, and justice agencies.
- Disseminates knowledge to many audiences.

As part of its standard development activities, NIJ serves as the executive agent for the Interagency Board for Equipment Standardization and Interoperability (IAB). The IAB has developed a set of priorities for standards for equipment to be used by first responders to critical incidents, including terrorist incidents relating to chemical, biological, nuclear, radiological, and explosive weapons. In particular, the development of chemical and biological defense equipment guides for the emergency first responder community is a high priority of NIJ.

The Office of Law Enforcement Standards (OLES) of the National Institute of Standards and Technology (NIST) furnishes technical support to NIJ in the development of standards. OLES subjects existing equipment to laboratory testing and evaluation and conducts research leading to the development of national standards, user guides, and technical reports.

This document covers research conducted by OLES under the sponsorship of NIJ. Other NIJ documents developed by OLES cover protective clothing and equipment, communications systems, emergency equipment, investigative aids, security systems, vehicles, weapons, analytical techniques, and standard reference materials used by the forensic community.

Technical comments and suggestions concerning this guide are invited from all interested parties. They may be addressed to the Office of Law Enforcement Standards, National Institute of Standards and Technology, 100 Bureau Drive, Stop 8102, Gaithersburg, MD 20899–8102.

Sarah V. Hart, Director
National Institute of Justice

Contents

FOREWORD iii
COMMONLY USED SYMBOLS AND ABBREVIATIONS vi
ABOUT THIS GUIDE ix
1. INTRODUCTION 1
2. IDENTIFICATION OF PERSONAL PROTECTIVE EQUIPMENT 3
   2.1 Identification of New Equipment 3
   2.2 Vendor Contact 3
3. DATA FIELDS 5
   3.1 General Category 5
   3.2 Operational Parameters Category 7
   3.3 Physical Parameters Category 8
   3.4 Logistical Parameters Category 9
   3.5 Special Requirements Category 11
APPENDIX A—REFERENCES A–1
APPENDIX B—INDEX BY PERCUTANEOUS PROTECTIVE EQUIPMENT
   (APPAREL) IDENTIFICATION NUMBER B–1
APPENDIX C—INDEX BY PERCUTANEOUS PROTECTIVE EQUIPMENT
   (APPAREL) NAME C–1
APPENDIX D—INDEX BY PERCUTANEOUS PROTECTIVE EQUIPMENT
   (APPAREL) MANUFACTURER D–1
APPENDIX E—PERCUTANEOUS PROTECTIVE EQUIPMENT (APPAREL) DATA
   SHEETS E–1

COMMONLY USED SYMBOLS AND ABBREVIATIONS

A	ampere	h	hour	oz.	ounce
ac	alternating current	hf	high frequency	No.	number
AM	amplitude modulation	Hz	hertz	o.d.	outside diameter
cd	candela	i.d.	inside diameter	Ω	ohm
cm	centimeter	in	inch	p.	page
CP	chemically pure	IR	infrared	Pa	pascal
c/s	cycle per second	J	joule	pe	probable error
d	day	L	lambert	pp.	pages
dB	decibel	L	liter	ppm	parts per million
dc	direct current	lb	pound	qt	quart
°C	degree Celsius	lbf	pound-force	rad	radian
°F	degree Fahrenheit	lbf·in	pound-force inch	rf	radio frequency
dia	diameter	lm	lumen	rh	relative humidity
emf	electromotive force	ln	logarithm (base e)	s	second
eq	equation	log	logarithm (base 10)	SD	standard deviation
F	farad	M	molar	sec.	Section
fc	footcandle	m	meter	SWR	standing wave ratio
fig.	Figure	μ	micron	uhf	ultrahigh frequency
FM	frequency modulation	min	minute	UV	ultraviolet
ft	foot	mm	millimeter	V	volt
ft/s	foot per second	mph	miles per hour	vhf	very high frequency
g	acceleration	m/s	meter per second	W	watt
g	gram	mo	month	λ	wavelength
gal	gallon	N	newton	wk	week
gr	grain	N·m	newton meter	wt	weight
H	henry	nm	nanometer	yr	year

area=unit^2 (e.g., ft^2, in^2, etc.); volume=unit^3 (e.g., ft^3, m^3, etc.)

ACRONYMS SPECIFIC TO THIS DOCUMENT

ASTM	American Society for Testing and Materials	NIJ	National Institute of Justice
BW	Biological Warfare	NIOSH	National Institute for Occupational Safety and Health
CB	Chemical and Biological	NIST	National Institute of Standards and Technology
CBW	Chemical Biological Warfare	NATO	North Atlantic Treaty Organization
CPU	Collective Protective Undergarment	NBC	Nuclear, Biological, and Chemical
CW	Chemical Warfare	OSHA	Occupational Safety and Health Administration
DOD	Department of Defense	PAPR	Powered Air Purifying Respirator
DTAPS	Disposable Toxicological Agent Protective Suit	PF	Protection Factor
DPG	Dugway Proving Grounds	PICS	Personal Ice Cooling System
DRES	Defense Research Establishment Suffield	POL	Petroleum, Oils, and Lubricants
ECBE	Edgewood Chemical Biological Center, Aberdeen Proving Ground, MD	PPE	Personal Protective Equipment
EOD	Explosive Ordnance Disposal	PPV	Positive Pressure Ventilation
EPA	Environmental Protection Agency	PVC	Polyvinyl chloride
ERDEC	U.S. Army Edgewood Research, Development and Engineering Center	SBCCOM	U.S. Army Soldier and Biological Chemical Command
FBI	Federal Bureau of Investigation	SCBA	Self-Contained Breathing Apparatus
FR	Fire Resistant	STB	Super Tropical Bleach
HAZMAT	Hazardous Materials	TAP	Toxicological Agent Protective
IDLH	Immediately Dangerous to Life and Health	TICs	Toxic Industrial Chemicals
IAB	Interagency Board	TIMs	Toxic Industrial Materials
ITAR	International Traffic and Arms Regulations	TOP	Test Operating Procedure
NFPA	National Fire Protection Association	TSWG	Technical Support Working Group

PREFIXES (See ASTM E380)				**COMMON CONVERSIONS**	
d	deci (10^{-1})	da	deka (10)	0.30480 m = 1 ft	4.448222 N = 1 lbf
c	centi (10^{-2})	h	hecto (10^2)	25.4 mm = 1 in	1.355818 J = 1 ft·lbf
m	milli (10^{-3})	k	kilo (10^3)	0.4535924 kg = 1 lb	0.1129848 N m = 1 lbf·in
μ	micro (10^{-6})	M	mega (10^6)	0.06479891 g = 1 gr	14.59390 N/m = 1 lbf/ft
n	nano (10^{-9})	G	giga (10^9)	0.9463529 L = 1 qt	6894.757 Pa = 1 lbf/in^2
p	pico (10^{-12})	T	tera (10^{12})	3600000 J = 1 kW·hr	1.609344 km/h = 1 mph

psi = mm of Hg x (1.9339 x 10^{-2})
mm of Hg = psi x 51.71

Temperature: $T_C = (T_F - 32) \times 5/9$ Temperature: $T_F = (T_C \times 9/5) + 32$

ABOUT THIS GUIDE

The National Institute of Justice is the focal point for providing support to State and local law enforcement agencies in the development of counterterrorism technology and standards, including technology needs for chemical and biological defense. In recognizing the needs of State and local emergency first responders, the Office of Law Enforcement Standards (OLES) at the National Institute of Standards and Technology (NIST), supported by the National Institute of Justice, the Technical Support Working Group (TSWG), the U.S. Army Soldier and Biological Chemical Command, and the Interagency Board for Equipment Standardization and Interoperability (IAB), is developing chemical and biological defense equipment guides. The guides will focus on chemical and biological equipment in areas of detection, personal protection, decontamination, and communication. This document focuses specifically on assisting the emergency first responder community in the evaluation and purchase of personal protective equipment.

The long range plans are to: (1) subject existing personal protective equipment to laboratory testing and evaluation against a specified protocol, and (2) conduct research leading to the development of multiple series of documents, including national standards, user guides, and technical reports. It is anticipated that the testing, evaluation, and research processes will take several years to complete; therefore, the National Institute of Justice has developed this initial guide for the emergency first responder community in order to facilitate their evaluation and purchase of personal protective equipment.

In conjunction with this program, additional guides, as well as other documents, are being issued in the areas of chemical agent and toxic industrial material detection equipment, biological agent detection equipment, decontamination equipment, and communication equipment.

This Volume, IIc, of the *Guide for the Selection of Personal Protective Equipment for Emergency First Responders*, which focuses on percutaneous (skin) protection other than garments—herein referred to as apparel (e.g., hoods, labcoats, and gloves). It contains the information data sheets that were used to support the personal protective equipment evaluation detailed in Volume I. The compilation of data in Volume IIc is the result of the merger of several data acquisition methods used independently by NIST and TSWG.

The information contained in this guide has been obtained through literature searches and market surveys. The vendors were contacted multiple times during the preparation of this guide to ensure data accuracy. In addition, the information is supplemented with test data obtained from other sources (e.g., Department of Defense), if available. It should also be noted that the purpose of this guide is not to provide recommendations but rather to serve as a means to provide information to the reader to compare and contrast commercially available personal protective equipment. *Reference herein to any specific commercial products, processes, or services by trade name, trademark, manufacturer, or otherwise does not necessarily constitute or imply its endorsement, recommendation, or favoring by the United States Government. The information and statements contained in this guide shall not be used for the purposes of advertising, nor to imply the endorsement or recommendation of the United States Government.*

With respect to information provided in this guide, neither the United States Government nor any of its employees make any warranty, expressed or implied, including but not limited to the warranties of merchantability and fitness for a particular purpose. Further, neither the United States Government nor any of its employees assume any legal liability or responsibility for the accuracy, completeness, or usefulness of any information, apparatus, product, or process disclosed.

Technical comments, suggestions, and product updates are encouraged from interested parties. They may be addressed to the Office of Law Enforcement Standards, National Institute of Standards and Technology, 100 Bureau Drive, Stop 8102, Gaithersburg, MD 20899–8102. It is anticipated that this guide will be updated periodically.

Questions relating to the specific devices included in this document should be addressed directly to the proponent agencies or the equipment manufacturers. Contact information for each equipment item included in this guide can be found in this volume (Vol. IIc).

GUIDE FOR THE SELECTION OF PERSONAL PROTECTIVE EQUIPMENT FOR EMERGENCY FIRST RESPONDERS (PERCUTANEOUS PROTECTION—APPAREL)

This guide includes information intended to be useful to the emergency first responder community in the selection of personal protective equipment (PPE) that includes chemical and biological protective clothing and respiratory equipment for different applications. This Volume, IIc, of the *Guide for the Selection of Personal Protective Equipment for Emergency First Responders*, includes details on the 74 percutaneous protective items (apparel other than garments) that are referenced in Volume I.

1. INTRODUCTION

The *Guide for the Selection of Personal Protective Equipment for Emergency First Responders* includes information intended to be useful to the emergency first responder community in the selection of PPE (percutaneous and respiratory). Due to the large number of PPE items identified for the guide, the guide is separated into four volumes. Volume I serves as the selection tool for all PPE, while Volume IIa serves as a repository for the respiratory protective data sheets; Volume IIb serves as a repository for the percutaneous protective equipment (garments) data sheets, and Volume IIc serves as a repository for the percutaneous protective equipment (apparel) data sheets.

2. IDENTIFICATION OF PERSONAL PROTECTIVE EQUIPMENT

An extensive market survey was conducted to identify commercially available personal protective equipment. This market survey encompassed the assessment of past market surveys, identification of new equipment, and interaction with numerous equipment vendors.

2.1 Identification of New Equipment

A variety of sources were utilized to identify commercially available personal protective equipment, including a Commerce Business Daily (CBD) Announcement, literature searches, database searches, Internet searches, technical conferences, and technical contacts. These sources resulted in the identification of 74 percutaneous protective equipment items.

2.2 Vendor Contact

Vendors were contacted three separate times in order to obtain additional product information, as well as to finalize their specific equipment data for inclusion in the guide. An initial contact with vendors and manufacturers occurred the last quarter of 1999, when they received a facsimile or an electronic mail message that contained the definitions for the data fields. They were asked to supply information on vendor specific personal equipment items corresponding to the data field definitions.

The second contact occurred during the March/April 2000 time period in order to finalize the equipment data sheets and the information contained in the guide. This contact was conducted by facsimile and electronic mail. The vendors were given two weeks to review the information.

The third contact was made during February 2001. Each vendor received a facsimile or an electronic mail message that contained the data sheets for their specific equipment item(s), the selection factors that were developed to assist with the selection and purchase of the most appropriate equipment, and the results of the evaluation of the personal protective equipment against the selection factors. The vendors were asked to review the data sheets and tables for completeness and accuracy of the incorporated data. The vendors were given three weeks to review the information.

3. DATA FIELDS

Appendix E serves as a compendium of commercially available personal protective equipment. Each of the 74 identified percutaneous protective items is detailed within appendix E. Forty-nine data fields, as defined in this section, were used for providing information relating to the personal protective equipment. It is important to note that these data fields were developed using input from the emergency responder community.

The data fields are organized into the following five categories:

- General.
- Operational Parameters.
- Physical Parameters.
- Logistical.
- Special Requirements.

The remainder of this section defines each of the 49 data fields by category.

3.1 General Category

The General Category includes the following data fields:

1. Name.
2. ID #.
3. Technology.
4. Stock Number.
5. Protection Type.
6. Equipment Category.
7. Availability.
8. Current User.
9. Manufacturer.
10. Manufacturer Type.
11. Developer.
12. Source.
13. Certification.

Each of these data fields is defined in more detail in the remainder of this section.

3.1.1 Name

The Name data field is used to identify the name of the equipment.

3.1.2 ID

The ID # data field is for identification purposes only.

3.1.3 Technology

The Technology data field identifies the material or process by which a piece of equipment supplies protection from chemical and biological agents, nuclear particulates, and/or toxic industrial materials (TIMs). Percutaneous protection is generally afforded by material technologies (such as carbon sphere materials, selectively-permeable or semi-permeable materials) or finish/treatment or coating add-ons (such as a water-repellant coating, an electrostatic finish, or a reactive coating).

3.1.4 Stock Number

The Stock Number data field includes the stock identification or national stock number, if the item has one.

3.1.5 Protection Type

The Protection Type data field identifies whether the equipment provides percutaneous (skin) and/or respiratory protection.

3.1.6 Equipment Category

The Equipment Category data field identifies if the equipment is self-contained breathing apparatus (SCBA), powered air purifying respirator (PAPR), tethered air, and/or canister.

3.1.7 Availability

The Availability data field refers to how readily available a piece of equipment is (e.g., how long it takes to receive equipment upon purchasing) or availability status of the equipment (e.g., commercial availability).

3.1.8 Current User

The Current User data field is used to identify organizations that are currently using the piece of equipment.

3.1.9 Manufacturer

The Manufacturer data field indentifies the company that manufactured the piece of equipment (to include the name, address, telephone number, and point-of-contact (POC)).

3.1.10 Manufacturer Type

The Manufacturer Type data field indicates whether the manufacturer is domestic or foreign.

3.1.11 Developer

The Developer data field identifies the organization that developed the item. This may be relevant when the developer is the government and the responsible technical agency may need to be identified.

3.1.12 Source

The Source data field indicates where the equipment information was obtained. Potential sources include past market surveys and Internet web sites.

3.1.13 Certification

The Certification data field identifies the agency certifying the system for use (i.e., OSHA, NIOSH, NFPA, etc.), if any.

3.2 Operational Parameters Category

The Operational Parameters Category includes the following five data fields:

1. Chemical Warfare (CW) Agents Protection.
2. Biological Warfare (BW) Agents Protection.
3. Toxic Industrial Materials (TIMs) Protection.
4. Duration of Protection.
5. Recommended Use(s).

Each of these data fields is defined in more detail in the remainder of this section.

3.2.1 Chemical Warfare (CW) Agents Protection

The Chemical Warfare Agents Protection data field indicates the type of chemical warfare (CW) agent. The most common types of classic CW agents are the nerve and blister agents. Nerve agents include GA (Tabun), GB (Sarin), GD (Soman), GF, and VX. Blister agents include H and HD (Sulfur Mustards), HN (Nitrogen Mustard), and L (Lewisite).

3.2.2 Biological Warfare (BW) Agents Protection

The Biological Warfare (BW) Agents Protection data field indicates the type of biological warfare (BW) agent. Classical BW agents include bacteria (Anthrax), rickettsia (Typhus), toxins (Botulinum Toxin), and viruses (Q Fever).

3.2.3 Toxic Industrial Materials (TIMs) Protection

The Toxic Industrial Materials (TIMs) Protection data field indicates the type of toxic industrial material (TIM) agent. TIMs are used in a variety of settings such as manufacturing facilities, maintenance areas, and storage areas. TIMs are further characterized by using a high, medium, or low hazard index. Examples of TIMs are ammonia, carbon monoxide, chlorine, hydrogen cyanide, phosgene, and mineral acids (i.e., hydrochloric acid, sulfuric acid, and nitric acid).

3.2.4 Duration of Protection

The Duration of Protection data field indicates the amount of time the equipment provides adequate protection. Since duration varies depending on the concentration of agent, type of agent, and environmental conditions, duration will be given with respect to specific conditions.

3.2.5 Recommended Use(s)

The Recommended Use(s) data field identifies the areas where the equipment is most likely to be used per vendor or manufacturer recommendation (e.g., tactical operations, and crisis management).

3.3 Physical Parameters Category

The Physical Parameters Category includes the following data fields:

1. Sizes Available.
2. Weight.
3. Package Size and Volume.
4. Power Requirements.
5. Material Type (Percutaneous).
6. Construction Type (Percutaneous).
7. Color.

Each of these data fields is defined in more detail in the remainder of this section.

3.3.1 Sizes Available

The Sizes Available data field provides available sizes for an item, to include both male and female when appropriate.

3.3.2 Weight

The Weight data field indicates the total weight of the equipment/system.

3.3.3 Package Size and Volume

The Package Size and Volume data field provides the external dimensions of the system when packaged (for storage and transportability).

3.3.4 Power Requirements

The Power Requirements data field indicates the type of power (ac, dc, etc.) required to operate the equipment. This category applies primarily to respiratory, respiratory support equipment, and heating/cooling systems.

3.3.5 Material Type (Percutaneous)

The Material Type data field refers to the material content of the suit and the level of impermeability (i.e., impermeable, selectively permeable, or permeable). Note if the protective clothing is fire retardant or contains thermoplastic material (could potentially burn the wearer).

3.3.6 Construction Type (Percutaneous)

The Construction Type data field indicates how seams are sealed. This data field applies primarily to percutaneous equipment.

3.3.7 Color

The Color data field indicates if equipment has camouflage capability (signature reduction). Color can help identify job type.

3.4 Logistical Parameters Category

The Logistical Parameters Category includes the following data fields:

1. Ease of Use.
2. Consumables.
3. Maintenance Requirements.
4. Shelf Life.
5. Transportability.
6. Operational Limitations.
7. Environmental Conditions.
8. Unit Cost.
9. Maintenance Cost.
10. Warranty.
11. Don/Doff Information.
12. Use/Reuse.
13. Launderability (Percutaneous).
14. Accessories.

Each of these data fields is defined in more detail in the remainder of this section.

3.4.1 Ease of Use

Ease of Use is the mobility and flexibility of an individual while wearing the equipment as well as the compatibility of the equipment with other equipment.

3.4.2 Consumables

Consumables are the supplies used during operation and storage. Examples of consumables are batteries, canisters, hoses, etc.

3.4.3 Maintenance Requirements

Maintenance Requirements are the services and parts required to keep the system at its peak operational readiness (e.g., preventative maintenance) and the frequency of required maintenance (e.g., after use, quarterly, and annually).

3.4.4 Shelf Life

Shelf Life is the length of time a piece of equipment can be stored before it needs to be replaced. Shelf life includes the recommended storage procedure and any factors that decrease shelf life (e.g., UV, and critical temperature).

3.4.5 Transportability

Transportability is the ability of the equipment to be transported, including any support equipment (e.g., respiratory equipment, and heating/cooling systems).

3.4.6 Operational Limitations

Operational Limitations refer to the length of time responders can safely work at various temperatures (i.e., 50 °F, 70 °F, and 90 °F) and the availability/compatibility of cooling systems to help manage heat stress.

3.4.7 Environmental Conditions

Environmental Conditions indicate whether the equipment is designed for use in all common outdoor weather conditions and climates (e.g., rain, snow, extreme temperatures, and humidity) or only under relatively controlled conditions.

3.4.8 Unit Cost

Unit Cost is the cost of a complete system, including support equipment and operating costs (i.e., consumables).

3.4.9 Maintenance Cost

Maintenance Cost is the cost required to maintain the system at its operational readiness. This cost will be based on equipment usage rates.

3.4.10 Warranty

The Warranty is the length of time a piece of equipment is guaranteed by the manufacturer, including the terms of the warranty (parts and labor).

3.4.11 Don/Doff Information

The Don/Doff Information indicates whether the system requires assistance for donning and/or doffing and the average time for this activity.

3.4.12 Use/Reuse

Use/Reuse indicates the need for any part of the equipment to be discarded after use or its ability to be reused. The data field includes the procedures used to decontaminate and/or dispose of used equipment.

3.4.13 Launderability (Percutaneous)

Launderability includes the laundering procedures that are safe for the item, including the number of times the suit can be laundered and remain efficacious. Also, launderability includes any special procedures needed for specific components.

3.4.14 Accessories

Accessories include those items that are provided with the basic equipment.

3.5 Special Requirements Category

The Special Requirements Category includes the following data fields:

1. Training Requirements.
2. Training Available.
3. Manuals Available.
4. Surveillance Testing Requirements.
5. Support Equipment.
6. Testing Information.
7. Applicable Regulations.
8. Health Hazards.
9. Communications Interface Capability.
10. EOD Compatibility.

Each of these data fields is defined in more detail in the remainder of this section.

3.5.1 Training Requirements

The Training Requirements data field refers to the amount of instruction time the operator needs to become proficient in using a piece of equipment.

3.5.2 Training Available

The Training Available data field refers to training available from the manufacturer. This includes any initial training and recertification training that is available.

3.5.3 Manuals Available

The Manuals Available data field indicates the types of manuals available from the manufacturer (e.g., user manuals, and training documentation).

3.5.4 Surveillance Testing Requirements

The Surveillance Testing Requirements data field specifies the testing required to keep a piece of equipment at its operational readiness (e.g., inspecting respiratory masks or suits for holes or tears).

3.5.5 Support Equipment

The Support Equipment data field refers to any additional equipment required to operate the primary unit.

3.5.6 Testing Information

The Testing Information data field includes any test data obtained from the manufacturer and other sources regarding any part of the equipment (e.g., validation testing including materials and ensemble testing such as abrasion, tear, wear, burst, and permeation testing).

3.5.7 Applicable Regulations

The Applicable Regulations data field includes any government and/or safety regulations that may apply to the possession, use, or storage of any part of the system.

3.5.8 Health Hazards

The Health Hazards data field identifies all materials that possess a potential health hazard.

3.5.9 Communications Interface Capability

The Communications Interface Capability data field refers to the ability of the personal protective equipment to interface with a communications system (network capability, hardwire capability, and RF communication).

3.5.10 EOD Compatibility

The EOD Compatibility data field is the ability of the equipment to be used with EOD systems (i.e., suits). For example, a CB protective suit and respirator are required to be worn with an EOD suit in a CB environment.

APPENDIX A—REFERENCES

APPENDIX A—REFERENCES

1. Armando S. Bevelacqua and Richard H. Stilp, *Terrorism Handbook for Operational Responders*, Emergency Film Group, Edgartown, MA, January 1998.

2. Robert E. Hunt, Timothy Hayes, and Warren B. Carroll, *Guidelines for Mass Casualty Decontamination During a Terrorist Chemical Agent Incident*, Battelle, Columbus, OH, September 1999.

3. A.K. Stuempfle, D.J. Howells, S.J. Armour, and C.A. Boulet, *International Task Force 25: Hazard from Industrial Chemicals Final Report*, Edgewood Research Development and Engineering Center, Aberdeen Proving Ground, MD, AD–B236562, ERDEC–SP–061, April 1998.

4. *Responding to a Biological or Chemical Threat: A Practical Guide*, U.S. Department of State, Bureau of Diplomatic Security, Washington, DC, 1996.

5. *2000 Emergency Response Guidebook, A Guidebook for First Responders During the Initial Phase of a Dangerous Goods/Hazardous Materials Incident*, U.S. Department of Transportation, Research and Special Programs Administration, Tempest Publishing, Alexandria, VA, January 2000.

6. *Potential Military Chemical/Biological Agents and Compounds*, FM 3–9, AFR 355–7; NAVFAC P–467, Army Chemical School, Ft. McClellan, AL, December 12, 1990.

7. *Guidelines for Incident Commander's Use of Firefighter Protective Ensemble (FFPE) with Self Contained Breathing Apparatus (SCBA) for Rescue Operations During a Terrorist Chemical Agent Incident*, U.S. Army Soldier and Biological Chemical Command (SBCCOM) Domestic Preparedness Chemical Team, Aberdeen Proving Ground, MD, April 30, 1999.

8. Richard B. Belmonte, *Tests of Level A Suits—Protection Against Chemical and Biological Warfare Agents and Simulants: Executive Summary*, Soldier and Biological Chemical Command (SBCCOM), SCBRD-EN, Aberdeen Proving Ground, MD, June 1998.

9. Robert S. Lindsay, *Test Results of Level B Suits to Challenge by Chemical and Biological Warfare Agents and Simulants: Summary Report*, Soldier and Biological Chemical Command (SBCCOM), AMSSB-REN, Aberdeen Proving Ground, MD, April 1999.

APPENDIX B—INDEX BY PERCUTANEOUS PROTECTIVE EQUIPMENT (APPAREL) IDENTIFICATION NUMBER

Index by Percutaneous Protective Equipment (Apparel) Identification Number

ID #	Percutaneous PPE (Apparel) Name	Manufacturer	Page E-#
1	Toxicological Agent Protective (TAP) Boot	Acton International Inc.	1
2	NBC Multi-Purpose Safety Boot	Acton International Inc.	3
3	Acton Basic NBC Overboot	Acton International Inc.	5
4	Acton Lightweight NBC Overboot	Acton International Inc.	7
5	CB Molded Glove With Liner	Acton International Inc.	9
6	Ansell Sol-Vex Gloves	Ansell Occupational Healthcare	11
7	Bata HazMat Boots	Bata Shoe Co., Inc.	13
8	Bata Boot/Shoe Covers	Bata Shoe Co., Inc.	15
9	Butyl Plus-NBC/Toxic Protective Glove	COMESEC Safety Inc.	17
10	Multi Plus-HazMat/Toxic Protective Glove	COMESEC Safety Inc	19
11	Chemical Biological Protective Sock	CA Fashion Inc.	21
12	Tyvek® Labcoat	DuPont Tyvek® Protective Apparel	23
13	Tyvek® Labcoat	DuPont Tyvek® Protective Apparel	26
14	Tyvek® Shirt	DuPont Tyvek® Protective Apparel	29
15	Tyvek® Labcoat	DuPont Tyvek® Protective Apparel	32
16	Tyvek® Labcoat	DuPont Tyvek® Protective Apparel	35
17	Tyvek® Pants	DuPont Tyvek® Protective Apparel	38
18	Tyvek® Hood	DuPont Tyvek® Protective Apparel	41
19	Tyvek® Hood	DuPont Tyvek® Protective Apparel	44
20	Tyvek® Hood	DuPont Tyvek® Protective Apparel	47
21	Tychem® QC Labcoat	DuPont Tyvek® Protective Apparel	50
22	Tychem® QC Shirt	DuPont Tyvek® Protective Apparel	53
23	Tychem® QC Pants	DuPont Tyvek® Protective Apparel	56
24	Tychem® QC Hood	DuPont Tyvek® Protective Apparel	59
25	Tychem® QC Hood	DuPont Tyvek® Protective Apparel	62
26	Tychem® SL Hood	DuPont Tyvek® Protective Apparel	65
27	Tychem® BR Hood/Vest	DuPont Tyvek® Protective Apparel	68
28	Tychem® TK Hood/Vest	DuPont Tyvek® Protective Apparel	71
29	Integrated Chemical Biological Protective Glove	Wells Lamont	74
30	NBC Gloves	Goetzloff GmbH	76
31	Eurolite NBC-Casualty Bag	Goetzloff GmbH	78
32	Eurolite NBC-Cover Poncho	Goetzloff GmbH	80

ID #	Percutaneous PPE (Apparel) Name	Manufacturer	Page E-#
33	Chemical Protective Butyl Rubber Gloves	Guardian Manufacturing Co.	82
34	Chemical Protective Butyl Rubber Gloves	Guardian Manufacturing Co.	84
35	Neoprene Gloves	Guardian Manufacturing Co.	86
36	NBC Casualty Bag	Irvin Aerospace Canada Ltd.	88
37	Kappler CPF 4 Bib Overall	Kappler Safety Group	90
38	Kappler CPF 4 Hood	Kappler Safety Group	93
39	Kappler CPF 4 Jacket	Kappler Safety Group	96
40	Lakeland Tychem® 10000 Level B Jacket	Lakeland Industries, Inc.	99
41	Lakeland Tychem® 10000 Level B Overalls	Lakeland Industries, Inc.	101
42	Lakeland Tychem® 10000 Level B Hood	Lakeland Industries, Inc.	103
43	Lakeland Tychem® 10000 Level B Apron	Lakeland Industries, Inc.	105
44	Lakeland Tyvek® QC Level B Jacket	Lakeland Industries, Inc.	107
45	Lakeland Tyvek® QC Level B Pants	Lakeland Industries, Inc.	109
46	Lakeland Tyvek® QC Level B Hood	Lakeland Industries, Inc.	111
47	Lakeland Tyvek® QC Level B Sleeves	Lakeland Industries, Inc.	113
48	Lakeland Tychem® SL Level B Hood	Lakeland Industries, Inc.	115
49	Lakeland Tychem® SL Level B Hood	Lakeland Industries, Inc.	117
50	Lakeland Tychem® SL Level B Apron	Lakeland Industries, Inc.	119
51	Lakeland Tychem® SL Level B Boots	Lakeland Industries, Inc.	121
52	Lakeland Tychem® SL Level B Sleeves	Lakeland Industries, Inc.	123
53	Lakeland Tychem® 9400 Level B Jacket/Pants	Lakeland Industries, Inc.	125
54	Lakeland Tychem® 9400 Level B Hood	Lakeland Industries, Inc.	127
55	Lakeland Tychem® 9400 Level B Hood	Lakeland Industries, Inc.	129
56	Lakeland Tychem® 9400 Level B Apron	Lakeland Industries, Inc.	131
57	Lakeland Tychem® 9400 Level B Sleeves	Lakeland Industries, Inc.	133
58	Lakeland Tychem® 9400 Level B Boot Covers	Lakeland Industries, Inc.	135
59	Chemical Protective Undergarment (CPU)	LANX Fabric Systems	137
60	Escape Jacket C/92F with optional Escape Hood	New Pac Safety AB	140
61	PONCHO NP/60	New Pac Safety AB	142
62	North Silver Shield Gloves	North	144
63	Rocky Shoes and Boots	Rocky Shoes and Boots, Inc.	146
64	Servus HZT Hazmat Knee Boot	Servus Firefighter Footwear	148

ID #	Percutaneous PPE (Apparel) Name	Manufacturer	Page E-#
65	Saratoga Chemical Protective Gloves	Tex-Shield, Inc.	150
66	Saratoga Chemical Protective Socks	Tex-Shield, Inc.	152
67	Saratoga Chemical Protective Undergarment	Tex-Shield, Inc.	154
68	Tingley Hazproof Overboot	Tingley Rubber Corporation	156
69	Weapons of Mass Destruction (WMD) Contamination Containment Bag	ILC Dover, Inc.	158
70	Chemical-Biological Eye/Respiratory Disposable (C-BERD) Hood/Mask	ILC Dover, Inc.	160
71	ILC Model 15 Cool Vest	ILC Dover, Inc.	162
72	ILC Model 19 Cool Vest	ILC Dover, Inc.	164
73	Personal Ice Cooling System (PICS)	GEOMET Technologies, Inc.	166
74	Flexi ICE Cold Vest	INTERSPIRO INC.	169

APPENDIX C—INDEX BY PERCUTANEOUS PROTECTIVE EQUIPMENT (APPAREL) NAME

Index by Percutaneous Protective Equipment (Apparel) Name

Percutaneous PPE (Apparel) Name	Manufacturer	ID #	Page E-#
Acton Basic NBC Overboot	Acton International Inc.	3	5
Acton Lightweight NBC Overboot	Acton International Inc.	4	7
Ansell Sol-Vex Gloves	Ansell Occupational Healthcare	6	11
Bata Boot/Shoe Covers	Bata Shoe Co., Inc.	8	15
Bata HazMat Boots	Bata Shoe Co., Inc.	7	13
Butyl Plus-NBC/Toxic Protective Glove	COMESEC Safety Inc.	9	17
CB Molded Glove With Liner	Acton International Inc.	5	9
Chemical Biological Protective Sock	CA Fashion Inc.	11	21
Chemical Protective Butyl Rubber Gloves	Guardian Manufacturing Co.	33	82
Chemical Protective Butyl Rubber Gloves	Guardian Manufacturing Co.	34	84
Chemical Protective Undergarment (CPU)	LANX Fabric Systems	59	137
Chemical-Biological Eye/Respiratory Disposable (C-BERD) Hood/Mask	ILC Dover, Inc.	70	160
Escape Jacket C/92F with optional Escape Hood	New Pac Safety AB	60	140
Eurolite NBC-Casualty Bag	Goetzloff GmbH	31	78
Eurolite NBC-Cover Poncho	Goetzloff GmbH	32	80
Flexi ICE Cold Vest	INTERSPIRO INC.	74	169
ILC Model 15 Cool Vest	ILC Dover, Inc.	71	162
ILC Model 19 Cool Vest	ILC Dover, Inc.	72	164
Integrated Chemical Biological Protective Glove	Wells Lamont	29	74
Kappler CPF 4 Bib Overall	Kappler Safety Group	37	90
Kappler CPF 4 Hood	Kappler Safety Group	38	93
Kappler CPF 4 Jacket	Kappler Safety Group	39	96
Lakeland Tychem® 10000 Level B Apron	Lakeland Industries, Inc.	43	110
Lakeland Tychem® 10000 Level B Hood	Lakeland Industries, Inc.	42	103
Lakeland Tychem® 10000 Level B Jacket	Lakeland Industries, Inc.	40	99
Lakeland Tychem® 10000 Level B Overalls	Lakeland Industries, Inc.	41	101
Lakeland Tychem® 9400 Level B Apron	Lakeland Industries, Inc.	56	131
Lakeland Tychem® 9400 Level B Boot Covers	Lakeland Industries, Inc.	58	135
Lakeland Tychem® 9400 Level B Hood	Lakeland Industries, Inc.	54	127

Percutaneous PPE (Apparel) Name	Manufacturer	ID #	Page E-#
Lakeland Tychem® 9400 Level B Hood	Lakeland Industries, Inc.	55	129
Lakeland Tychem® 9400 Level B Jacket/Pants	Lakeland Industries, Inc.	53	125
Lakeland Tychem® 9400 Level B Sleeves	Lakeland Industries, Inc.	57	133
Lakeland Tychem® SL Level B Apron	Lakeland Industries, Inc.	50	119
Lakeland Tychem® SL Level B Boots	Lakeland Industries, Inc.	51	121
Lakeland Tychem® SL Level B Hood	Lakeland Industries, Inc.	48	115
Lakeland Tychem® SL Level B Hood	Lakeland Industries, Inc.	49	117
Lakeland Tychem® SL Level B Sleeves	Lakeland Industries, Inc.	52	123
Lakeland Tyvek® QC Level B Hood	Lakeland Industries, Inc.	46	111
Lakeland Tyvek® QC Level B Jacket	Lakeland Industries, Inc.	44	107
Lakeland Tyvek® QC Level B Pants	Lakeland Industries, Inc.	45	109
Lakeland Tyvek® QC Level B Sleeves	Lakeland Industries, Inc.	47	113
Multi Plus-HazMat/Toxic Protective Glove	COMESEC Safety Inc.	10	19
NBC Casualty Bag	Irvin Aerospace Canada Ltd.	36	88
NBC Gloves	Goetzloff GmbH	30	76
NBC Multi-Purpose Safety Boot	Acton International Inc.	2	3
Neoprene Gloves	Guardian Manufacturing Co.	35	86
North Silver Shield Gloves	North	62	144
Personal Ice Cooling System (PICS)	GEOMET Technologies, Inc.	73	166
PONCHO NP/60	New Pac Safety AB	61	142
Rocky Shoes and Boots	Rocky Shoes and Boots, Inc.	63	146
Saratoga Chemical Protective Gloves	Tex-Shield, Inc.	65	150
Saratoga Chemical Protective Socks	Tex-Shield, Inc.	66	152
Saratoga Chemical Protective Undergarment	Tex-Shield, Inc.	67	154
Servus HZT Hazmat Knee Boot	Servus Firefighter Footwear	64	148
Tingley Hazproof Overboot	Tingley Rubber Corporation	68	156
Toxicological Agent Protective (TAP) Boot	Acton International Inc.	1	1
Tychem® BR Hood/Vest	DuPont Tyvek® Protective Apparel	27	68
Tychem® QC Hood	DuPont Tyvek® Protective Apparel	24	59
Tychem® QC Hood	DuPont Tyvek® Protective Apparel	25	62
Tychem® QC Labcoat	DuPont Tyvek® Protective Apparel	21	50
Tychem® QC Pants	DuPont Tyvek® Protective Apparel	23	56
Tychem® QC Shirt	DuPont Tyvek® Protective Apparel	22	53

Percutaneous PPE (Apparel) Name	Manufacturer	ID #	Page E-#
Tychem® SL Hood	DuPont Tyvek® Protective Apparel	26	65
Tychem® TK Hood/Vest	DuPont Tyvek® Protective Apparel	28	71
Tyvek® Hood	DuPont Tyvek® Protective Apparel	18	41
Tyvek® Hood	DuPont Tyvek® Protective Apparel	19	44
Tyvek® Hood	DuPont Tyvek® Protective Apparel	20	47
Tyvek® Labcoat	DuPont Tyvek® Protective Apparel	12	23
Tyvek® Labcoat	DuPont Tyvek® Protective Apparel	13	26
Tyvek® Labcoat	DuPont Tyvek® Protective Apparel	15	32
Tyvek® Labcoat	DuPont Tyvek® Protective Apparel	16	35
Tyvek® Pants	DuPont Tyvek® Protective Apparel	17	38
Tyvek® Shirt	DuPont Tyvek® Protective Apparel	14	29
Weapons of Mass Destruction (WMD) Contamination Containment Bag	ILC Dover, Inc.	69	158

APPENDIX D—INDEX BY PERCUTANEOUS PROTECTIVE EQUIPMENT (APPAREL) MANUFACTURER

Index by Percutaneous Protective Equipment (Apparel) Manufacturer

Manufacturer	Percutaneous PPE (Apparel) Name	ID #	Page E-#
Acton International Inc.	Acton Basic NBC Overboot	3	5
Acton International Inc.	Acton Lightweight NBC Overboot	4	7
Acton International Inc.	CB Molded Glove With Liner	5	9
Acton International Inc.	NBC Multi-purpose Safety Boot	2	3
Acton International Inc.	Toxicological Agent Protective (TAP) Boot	1	1
Ansell Occupational Healthcare	Ansell Sol-Vex Gloves	6	11
Bata Shoe Co., Inc.	Bata Boot/Shoe Covers	8	15
Bata Shoe Co., Inc.	Bata HazMat Boots	7	13
CA Fashion Inc.	Chemical Biological Protective Sock	11	21
COMESEC Safety Inc.	Multi Plus-HazMat/Toxic Protective Glove	10	19
COMESEC Safety Inc.	Butyl Plus-NBC/Toxic Protective Glove	9	17
DuPont Tyvek® Protective Apparel	Tychem® BR Hood/Vest	27	68
DuPont Tyvek® Protective Apparel	Tychem® QC Hood	24	59
DuPont Tyvek® Protective Apparel	Tychem® QC Hood	25	62
DuPont Tyvek® Protective Apparel	Tychem® QC Labcoat	21	50
DuPont Tyvek® Protective Apparel	Tychem® QC Pants	23	56
DuPont Tyvek® Protective Apparel	Tychem® QC Shirt	22	53
DuPont Tyvek® Protective Apparel	Tychem® SL Hood	26	65
DuPont Tyvek® Protective Apparel	Tychem® TK Hood/Vest	28	71
DuPont Tyvek® Protective Apparel	Tyvek® Hood	18	41
DuPont Tyvek® Protective Apparel	Tyvek® Hood	19	44
DuPont Tyvek® Protective Apparel	Tyvek® Hood	20	47
DuPont Tyvek® Protective Apparel	Tyvek® Labcoat	12	23
DuPont Tyvek® Protective Apparel	Tyvek® Labcoat	13	26
DuPont Tyvek® Protective Apparel	Tyvek® Labcoat	15	32
DuPont Tyvek® Protective Apparel	Tyvek® Labcoat	16	35
DuPont Tyvek® Protective Apparel	Tyvek® Pants	17	38
DuPont Tyvek® Protective Apparel	Tyvek® Shirt	14	29
GEOMET Technologies, Inc.	Personal Ice Cooling System (PICS)	73	166
Goetzloff GmbH	Eurolite NBC-Casualty Bag	31	78
Goetzloff GmbH	Eurolite NBC-Cover Poncho	32	80
Goetzloff GmbH	NBC Gloves	30	76

Manufacturer	Percutaneous PPE (Apparel) Name	ID #	Page E–#
Guardian Manufacturing Co.	Chemical Protective Butyl Rubber Gloves	33	82
Guardian Manufacturing Co.	Chemical Protective Butyl Rubber Gloves	34	84
Guardian Manufacturing Co.	Neoprene Gloves	35	88
ILC Dover, Inc.	Chemical-Biological Eye/Respiratory Disposable (C-BERD) Hood/Mask	70	160
ILC Dover, Inc.	ILC Model 15 Cool Vest	71	162
ILC Dover, Inc.	ILC Model 19 Cool Vest	72	164
ILC Dover, Inc.	Weapons of Mass Destruction (WMD) Contamination Containment Bag	69	158
INTERSPIRO INC.	Flexi ICE Cold Vest	74	169
Irvin Aerospace Canada Ltd.	NBC Casualty Bag	36	93
Kappler Safety Group	Kappler CPF 4 Bib Overall	37	90
Kappler Safety Group	Kappler CPF 4 Hood	38	93
Kappler Safety Group	Kappler CPF 4 Jacket	39	96
Lakeland Industries, Inc.	Lakeland Tychem® 10000 Level B Apron	43	110
Lakeland Industries, Inc.	Lakeland Tychem® 10000 Level B Hood	42	103
Lakeland Industries, Inc.	Lakeland Tychem® 10000 Level B Jacket	40	99
Lakeland Industries, Inc.	Lakeland Tychem® 10000 Level B Overalls	41	101
Lakeland Industries, Inc.	Lakeland Tychem® 9400 Level B Apron	56	131
Lakeland Industries, Inc.	Lakeland Tychem® 9400 Level B Boot Covers	58	135
Lakeland Industries, Inc.	Lakeland Tychem® 9400 Level B Hood	54	127
Lakeland Industries, Inc.	Lakeland Tychem® 9400 Level B Hood	55	129
Lakeland Industries, Inc.	Lakeland Tychem® 9400 Level B Jacket/Pants	53	125
Lakeland Industries, Inc.	Lakeland Tychem® 9400 Level B Sleeves	57	133
Lakeland Industries, Inc.	Lakeland Tychem® SL Level B Apron	50	119
Lakeland Industries, Inc.	Lakeland Tychem® SL Level B Boots	51	121
Lakeland Industries, Inc.	Lakeland Tychem® SL Level B Hood	48	115
Lakeland Industries, Inc.	Lakeland Tychem® SL Level B Hood	49	117
Lakeland Industries, Inc.	Lakeland Tychem® SL Level B Sleeves	52	123
Lakeland Industries, Inc.	Lakeland Tyvek® QC Level B Hood	46	111
Lakeland Industries, Inc.	Lakeland Tyvek® QC Level B Jacket	44	107
Lakeland Industries, Inc.	Lakeland Tyvek® QC Level B Pants	45	109
Lakeland Industries, Inc.	Lakeland Tyvek® QC Level B Sleeves	47	113

Manufacturer	Percutaneous PPE (Apparel) Name	ID #	Page E-#
LANX Fabric Systems	Chemical Protective Undergarment (CPU)	59	137
New Pac Safety AB	Escape Jacket C/92F with optional Escape Hood	60	140
New Pac Safety AB	PONCHO NP/60	61	142
North	North Silver Shield Gloves	62	144
Rocky Shoes and Boots, Inc.	Rocky Shoes and Boots	63	146
Servus Firefighter Footwear	Servus HZT Hazmat Knee Boot	64	148
Tex-Shield, Inc.	Saratoga Chemical Protective Gloves	65	150
Tex-Shield, Inc.	Saratoga Chemical Protective Socks	66	152
Tex-Shield, Inc.	Saratoga Chemical Protective Undergarment	67	154
Tingley Rubber Corporation	Tingley Hazproof Overboot	68	156
Wells Lamont	Integrated Chemical Biological Protective Glove	29	74

APPENDIX E—PERCUTANEOUS PROTECTIVE EQUIPMENT (APPAREL) DATA SHEETS

Personal Protective Equipment (Percutaneous—Apparel)

General

Name	*Toxicological Agent Protective (TAP) Boot*
Item # 1	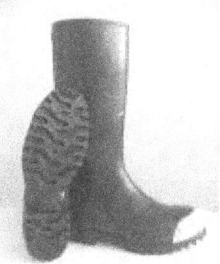
Technology	Extruded butyl material, hand assembled
Stock Number	8430–00–820–6301
Protection Type	NBC Resistant—24 h
Equipment Category	Footwear
Availability	In production
Current User(s)	U.S DOD and clean-up teams
Manufacturer	Acton International Inc. 881 Landry Acton Vale, Quebec J0H 1A0 450–546–2776 (Tel) 450–546–3735 (Fax)
Manufacturer Type	Acton International Inc.
Developer	Natick (Acton International Inc.)
Source	Acton International Inc.
Certification	Not applicable

Operational Parameters

Chemical Warfare (CW) Agents Protected Against	All known agents
Biological Warfare (BW) Agents Protected Against	All known agents
Toxic Industrial (TIMs) Protected Against	Not applicable
Duration of Protection	24 h (8 h U.S. Specification (Spec.) Requirements)
Recommended Use(s)	Clean-up operations, at incinerators, and toxic area clean-up

Physical Parameters

Sizes Available	5 through 17
Weight	5.6 lb per pair
Package Size and Volume	23 in x 1 in x 15 in
Power Requirements	Not applicable

Material Type	Butyl
Construction Type	Hand-assembled
Color	Black, yellow toe
Logistical Parameters	
Ease of Use	Not applicable
Consumables	Not applicable
Maintenance Requirements	Not applicable
Shelf Life	5 yr to 10 yr
Transportability	Not applicable
Operational Limitations	Not applicable
Environmental Conditions	-24 °F to 95 °F
Unit Cost	$75
Maintenance Cost	Not applicable
Warranty	1 yr
Don/Doff Information	Over sock
Use/Reuse	Can be reused
Launderability	Soap and water
Accessories	Not applicable
Special Requirements	
Training Requirements	Not applicable
Training Available	Not applicable
Manuals Available	Not applicable
Surveillance Testing Requirements	Not applicable
Support Equipment	Not applicable
Testing Information	CW test reports available (to 8 h requirement)
Applicable Regulations	Not applicable
Health Hazards	Not applicable
Communications Interface Capability	Not applicable
EOD Compatibility	Steel toe

General

Name *NBC Multi-Purpose Safety Boot*

Item # 2

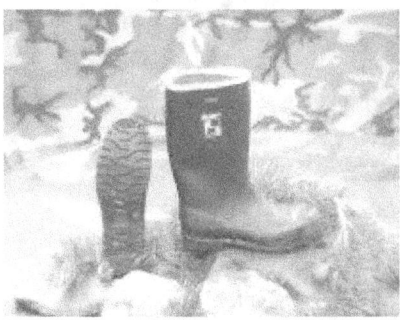

Technology Multi-layer polymer laminated with a nitrile chloroprene blend layer. Removable felt antistatic liner. Hand-assembled rubber footwear.

Stock Number Not specified

Protection Type 24 h NBC protection, meets EC requirements for firefighting boots (EN345–2: 1997). Steel toe, steel plate, and antistatic footwear

Equipment Category Footwear

Availability In production

Current User(s) Raddningsverket (SRV)
Sweden

Manufacturer Acton International Inc.
881 Landry
Acton Vale, Quebec
J0H 1A0
450–546–2776 (Tel)
450–546–3735 (Fax)

Manufacturer Type Foreign

Developer Acton International Inc.

Source Acton International Inc.

Certification EN 345–2: 1997

Operational Parameters

Chemical Warfare (CW) Agents Protected Against All known agents

Biological Warfare (BW) Agents Protected Against All known agents

Toxic Industrial (TIMs) Protected Against POL (oil, fuel)

Duration of Protection 24 h

Recommended Use(s) Clean-up, construction, firefighting, oilspills, and NBC activities

Physical Parameters

Sizes Available 38 to 46 (French Point)

Weight 5 lb per pair size 43 (9)

Package Size and Volume Each pair is in a bag; 5 to 7 pairs per box depending on boot size; box dimensions are 24 in x 16 in x 16 in

Power Requirements Not applicable

Material Type	Butyl rubber layer, laminated with a nitrile chloroprene blend layer
Construction Type	Hand-assembled, extruded and calandered rubber, and autoclave cured
Color	Black
Logistical Parameters	
Ease of Use	Not applicable
Consumables	Not applicable
Maintenance Requirements	Not applicable
Shelf Life	10 yr to 15 yr
Transportability	Not applicable
Operational Limitations	Not applicable
Environmental Conditions	-4 °F to 95 °F
Unit Cost	$65
Maintenance Cost	Not applicable
Warranty	1 yr
Don/Doff Information	Over the sock (pull on)
Use/Reuse	Not applicable
Launderability	Soap and water
Accessories	Removable lining
Special Requirements	
Training Requirements	Not applicable
Training Available	Not applicable
Manuals Available	Not applicable
Surveillance Testing Requirements	Not applicable
Support Equipment	Not applicable
Testing Information	CW test report from FOA Sweden available
Applicable Regulations	Not applicable
Health Hazards	Not applicable
Communications Interface Capability	Not applicable
EOD Compatibility	Anti-static, steel toe

General
Name — *Acton Basic NBC Overboot*
Item # 3

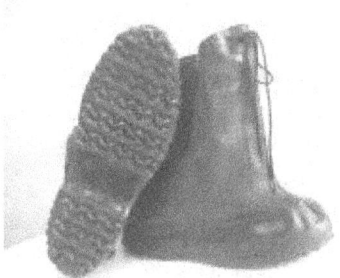

Technology	Extruded butyl compounded upper, lace closure at top
Stock Number	Not specified
Protection Type	24 h NBC protection and static
Equipment Category	Footwear, hand-assembled, and rubber footwear
Availability	Developed
Current User(s)	None: New inexpensive product being introduced in Europe
Manufacturer	Acton International Inc. 881 Landry Acton Vale, Quebec J0H 1A0 450–546–2776 (Tel) 450–546–3735 (Fax)
Manufacturer Type	Foreign
Developer	Acton International Inc.
Source	Acton International Inc.
Certification	Not applicable

Operational Parameters

Chemical Warfare (CW) Agents Protected Against	All known CW agents
Biological Warfare (BW) Agents Protected Against	All known CW agents
Toxic Industrial (TIMs) Protected Against	Not applicable
Duration of Protection	24 h
Recommended Use(s)	In conjunction with NBC suits in theatres of operation requiring full protection

Physical Parameters

Sizes Available	XS, S, M, L, XL, and XXL (covers primary footwear sizes 4 to 15)
Weight	2.2 lb per pair
Package Size and Volume	Various
Power Requirements	Not applicable
Material Type	Butyl rubber

Construction Type	Extruded butyl compounded upper, lace closure at top. Hand-assembled.
Color	Black
Logistical Parameters	
Ease of Use	Not applicable
Consumables	Not applicable
Maintenance Requirements	Not applicable
Shelf Life	10 yr to 15 yr
Transportability	Not applicable
Operational Limitations	Not applicable
Environmental Conditions	-31 °F to 122 °F
Unit Cost	$20
Maintenance Cost	Not applicable
Warranty	1 yr
Don/Doff Information	Over primary footwear
Use/Reuse	Can be decontaminated (liquid)
Launderability	Soap and water
Accessories	Elastic loop fasteners
Special Requirements	
Training Requirements	Not applicable
Training Available	Not applicable
Manuals Available	Not applicable
Surveillance Testing Requirements	Not applicable
Support Equipment	Not applicable
Testing Information	CW and physical property test reports can be made available
Applicable Regulations	Not applicable
Health Hazards	Not applicable
Communications Interface Capability	Not applicable
EOD Compatibility	Anti-static

General

Name *Acton Lightweight NBC Overboot*
Item # 4

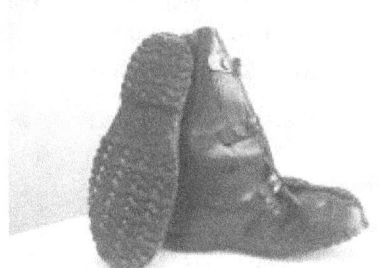

Technology — Extruded butyl material, elastic loop closure system, anti-static, snug fit, and can be decontaminated. Hand-assembled, extruded rubber.

Stock Number — 8430–99–869–0394 to 0399; 8430–99–869–0538 to 0543

Protection Type — NBC Resistant - greater than 24 h, can be decontaminated

Equipment Category — Footwear

Availability — In use worldwide - some stock maintained, large order produced per order

Current User(s) — United Kingdom (UK) MOD, Canadian DND, Australian DOD, New Zealand Armed Forces, OPCW, Kuwait MOD, and the National Guard

Manufacturer — Acton International Inc.
881 Landry
Acton Vale, Quebec
J0H 1A0
450–546–2776 (Tel)
450–546–3735 (Fax)

Manufacturer Type — Foreign

Developer — Acton International Inc.

Source — Acton International Inc.

Certification — Not applicable

Operational Parameters

Chemical Warfare (CW) Agents Protected Against — All known agents

Biological Warfare (BW) Agents Protected Against — All known agents

Toxic Industrial (TIMs) Protected Against — Not applicable

Duration of Protection — >24 h

Recommended Use(s) — All applications dealing with CW agents, armed forces, special operations, labs, and inspection teams.

Physical Parameters

Sizes Available — 6 sizes: XS, S, M, L, XL, and XXL. Fit over primary sizes 4 to 15.

Weight — 2.6 lb per pair average size (M)

Package Size and Volume — Bag: 1.6 in x 0.6 in x 0.3 in max (1pair per bag)
Carton: 17 in x 13 in x 13 in (10 pair per carton)

Power Requirements	Not applicable
Material Type	Butyl, extruded
Construction Type	Hand-assembled. Extruded butyl material, elastic loop closure system, anti-static, snug fit, and can be decontaminated.
Color	Black

Logistical Parameters

Ease of Use	Not applicable
Consumables	Not applicable
Maintenance Requirements	Not applicable
Shelf Life	10 yr to 15 yr
Transportability	Not applicable
Operational Limitations	Not applicable
Environmental Conditions	-31 °F to 122 °F
Unit Cost	$28 to $32 depending on features
Maintenance Cost	Not applicable
Warranty	1 yr
Don/Doff Information	Over primary footwear
Use/Reuse	Can be decontaminated
Launderability	Soap and water
Accessories	Elastic loops

Special Requirements

Training Requirements	Not applicable
Training Available	Not applicable
Manuals Available	Not applicable
Surveillance Testing Requirements	Not applicable
Support Equipment	Not applicable
Testing Information	CW and physical property test report available
Applicable Regulations	Not applicable
Health Hazards	Not applicable
Communications Interface Capability	Not applicable
EOD Compatibility	Anti-static

General
Name — *CB Molded Glove With Liner*
Item # 5

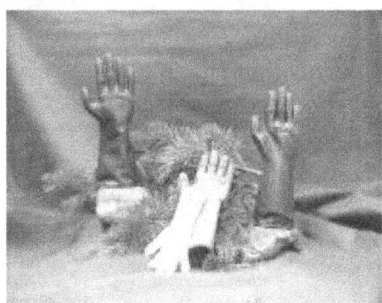

Technology	Accurate thin molding, excellent fit
Stock Number	Not specified
Protection Type	CW resistant; also POL resistant and antistatic models available
Equipment Category	Gloves, molded
Availability	Final prototypes - May 2000
Current User(s)	Not applicable—new Technology introduced in 2000
Manufacturer	Acton International Inc. 881 Landry Acton Vale, Quebec J0H 1A0 450–546–2776 (Tel) 450–546–3735 (Fax)
Manufacturer Type	Foreign
Developer	Acton International Inc., and Defense Research Establishment Suffield (DRES)
Source	Acton International Inc.
Certification	Not applicable

Operational Parameters

Chemical Warfare (CW) Agents Protected Against	All known agents
Biological Warfare (BW) Agents Protected Against	All known agents
Toxic Industrial (TIMs) Protected Against	One model will be POL resistant
Duration of Protection	12 h to 24 h depending on polymer and thickness
Recommended Use(s)	With all types of NBC Suits, for medical work, in labs, and in military theaters

Physical Parameters

Sizes Available	7 sizes (S, M, M-Narrow, L, L-Narrow, XL, and XL-Narrow)
Weight	200 g/pair, glove, and liner
Package Size and Volume	1 pair per bag, unknown quantity per box
Power Requirements	Not applicable
Material Type	Butyl or nitrile/chloroprene

Construction Type	Molded
Color	Black, other colors can be manufactured for large orders
Logistical Parameters	
Ease of Use	Not applicable
Consumables	Not applicable
Maintenance Requirements	Not applicable
Shelf Life	10 yr to 15 yr
Transportability	Not applicable
Operational Limitations	Not applicable
Environmental Conditions	5 °F to 122 °F
Unit Cost	$8 to $20 per pair
Maintenance Cost	Not applicable
Warranty	1 yr
Don/Doff Information	Molded glove can be worn directly over hand or with its liner
Use/Reuse	Not applicable
Launderability	Soap and water
Accessories	Coolmax, lycra removable liner
Special Requirements	
Training Requirements	Not applicable
Training Available	Not applicable
Manuals Available	Not applicable
Surveillance Testing Requirements	Not applicable
Support Equipment	Not applicable
Testing Information	CW test information shall be available in 2nd half of year 2000
Applicable Regulations	Not applicable
Health Hazards	Not applicable
Communications Interface Capability	Not applicable
EOD Compatibility	Snug fit, antistatic model

General
Name — *Ansell Sol-Vex Gloves*
Item # 6
Picture Not Available

Technology — Nitrile polymer
Stock Number — Ansell Stock No. 37–175
Protection Type — Percutaneous
Equipment Category — Gloves
Availability — Commercially available
Current User(s) — Industrial end-users worldwide
Manufacturer — Ansell Occupational Healthcare
1300 Walnut Street
Coshocton, OH 43812
740–622–4311(Tel)
800–800–0444 (Tel)
800–800–0445 (Fax)
Manufacturer Type — Global
Developer — Ansell Occupational Healthcare
Source — Internet: http://www.r-e-c.com
Response Equipment Co., a subsidiary of EAI Corporation
Certification — ASTM standards; FDA—accepted materials

Operational Parameters
Chemical Warfare (CW) Agents Protected Against — Not recommended

Biological Warfare (BW) Agents Protected Against — Not recommended

Toxic Industrial (TIMs) Protected Against — High level of protection vs. petroleum solvents, many caustics and acids, animal fats, and edible oils. Fair protection vs. aromatic solvents and esters. Not recommended for ketones.

Duration of Protection — Depends on concentration, time/length of exposure, other application factors. See Manufacturer's Guide CRG-CG-Rev. 9–98.

Recommended Use(s) — Chemical resistance

Physical Parameters
Sizes Available — 6–6 1/2 or 7–7 1/2 to 11; lengths: 13 in, 15 in, and 18 in
Weight — Depends on size
Package Size and Volume — 1.77 ft^3 full case (144 pair per full case)
Power Requirements — None
Material Type — Nitrile polymer
Construction Type — Not specified

Color	Green

Logistical Parameters

Ease of Use	Highly flexible
Consumables	None
Maintenance Requirements	None
Shelf Life	Indefinite when stored in original wrapper
Transportability	Not applicable
Operational Limitations	Not specified
Environmental Conditions	Normal indoor and outdoor temperatures
Unit Cost	Price set by distributors
Maintenance Cost	None
Warranty	Guaranteed against defects in workmanship and materials, and subject to proper storage and handling
Don/Doff Information	No assistance necessary
Use/Reuse	Reusable
Launderability	Not recommended
Accessories	None

Special Requirements

Training Requirements	None
Training Available	None required
Manuals Available	None required
Surveillance Testing Requirements	Visual inspection before and after each use
Support Equipment	None
Testing Information	Not specified
Applicable Regulations	Not specified
Health Hazards	Contains no natural rubber latex
Communications Interface Capability	Not applicable
EOD Compatibility	Not specified

General

Name — *Bata HazMat Boots*
Item # 7

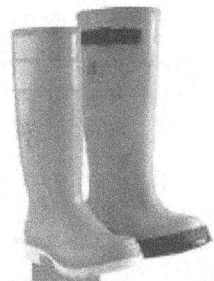

Technology	Nonabsorbent polyester lining
Stock Number	87012—16 in, steel toe boot with Ultragrip® Sipe Sole 87050—17 in, strapper with self-cleaning cleated sole
Protection Type	Percutaneous
Equipment Category	Boots (HazMat)—16 in oversock, kneeboots
Availability	Not specified
Current User(s)	Not specified
Manufacturer	Bata Shoe Co., Inc. 4501 Pulaski Highway Belcamp, MD 21017 POC: Joseph W. Diem 800–365–2282 (Tel) 410–272–2000 Ext.117 (Tel)
Manufacturer Type	Manufacturer of polyvinyl chloride (PVC) work boots - Industrial polymer safety footwear
Developer	Bata Shoe Co., Inc.
Source	Bata Shoe Co., Inc.
Certification	NFPA 199, 2000 Edition, Chemical Permeation Resistance Requirements and Flammability Resistance Tests; ANSI Std Z41–PR, Z41 Pt99 I/75 C/75; and CSA Std Z195 M92 Grade 1

Operational Parameters

Chemical Warfare (CW) Agents Protected Against	Certified for chemical terrorism incidents for the following CW agents: Cyanogen chloride, lewisite, sarin, V-agents, and sulphur mustard, distilled
Biological Warfare (BW) Agents Protected Against	Certified for biological terrorism incidents, protects against some biological agents
Toxic Industrial (TIMs) Protected Against	Protects against a variety of TIMs
Duration of Protection	Varies with chemical, most greater than 6 h
Recommended Use(s)	HazMat

Physical Parameters

Sizes Available	Men's full sizes 6 to 15
Weight	Not specified
Package Size and Volume	Not specified

Power Requirements	None
Material Type	Nonabsorbent polyester lining
Construction Type	Steel toe, full steel mid-sole, and seamless construction
Color	Chemical, green upper with yellow soles

Logistical Parameters

Ease of Use	Not specified
Consumables	None
Maintenance Requirements	The integrity and safety of the boot product can be maintained through proper cleaning, storage, and inspection procedures. Repairs are not recommended.
Shelf Life	Shelf life is diminished under storage conditions such as high temperature and humidity, over exposure to sunlight, vapors or cross contamination of other garments, and storage containers or tools
Transportability	Not applicable
Operational Limitations	Not recommended that the boots be worn in chemical depths that might result in the chemical being splashed into the top of the boot
Environmental Conditions	Protects in normal environments
Unit Cost	Not specified
Maintenance Cost	None
Warranty	Reference the Bata product literature for any warranty information
Don/Doff Information	No assistance necessary
Use/Reuse	Reusable
Launderability	Use only a mild soap solution to clean the boots, avoid chemical cleaning agents that may attack the boot product, avoid using unless thoroughly cleaned and tried
Accessories	Nonabsorbent polyester lining

Special Requirements

Training Requirements	None
Training Available	None required
Manuals Available	None required
Surveillance Testing Requirements	Visual inspection before and after each use
Support Equipment	Recommended undergarments: A minimum of cotton socks
Testing Information	Chemical permeation tests in accordance with ASTMF–739; flammability resistance test in accordance with Federal Test Method 5903.1
Applicable Regulations	Not specified
Health Hazards	None
Communications Interface Capability	Not specified
EOD Compatibility	Not specified

General
Name — *Bata Boot/Shoe Covers*
Item # 8

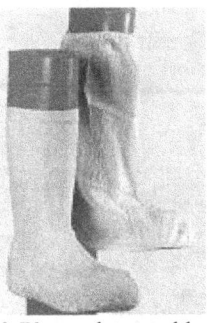

Technology	0.70 mm latex rubber
Stock Number	97590/97591
Protection Type	Percutaneous
Equipment Category	Boots/shoe covers
Availability	Available from stock
Current User(s)	Hazardous materials handling
Manufacturer	Bata Shoe Co., Inc. 4501 Pulaski Highway Belcamp, MD 21017 POC: Joseph W. Diem 800–365–2282 (Tel) 410–272–2000 Ext. 117 (Tel)
Manufacturer Type	Manufacturer of PVC work boots - Industrial polymer safety footwear
Developer	Bata Shoe Co., Inc.
Source	Bata Shoe Co., Inc.
Certification	NFPA 199, 2000 Edition, Chemical Permeation Resistance Requirements and Flammability Resistance Tests

Operational Parameters

Chemical Warfare (CW) Agents Protected Against	Chemical terrorism incidents with cyanogen chloride, lewisite, sarin, V-agents, and sulphur mustard, distilled
Biological Warfare (BW) Agents Protected Against	Biological terrorism incidents, protects against some biological agents
Toxic Industrial (TIMs) Protected Against	Protects against a variety of TIMs
Duration of Protection	Varies with chemical, most greater than 6 h
Recommended Use(s)	Protection from a broad range of materials, both hazardous and non-hazardous

Physical Parameters

Sizes Available	M to 2XXL
Weight	Lightweight
Package Size and Volume	Not specified
Power Requirements	None
Material Type	Latex rubber

Construction Type	None required
Color	Yellow

Logistical Parameters

Ease of Use	Slip-on/slip-off
Consumables	None
Maintenance Requirements	None
Shelf Life	None required
Transportability	Not applicable
Operational Limitations	Not specified
Environmental Conditions	Protects in normal environments
Unit Cost	Not specified
Maintenance Cost	None
Warranty	Not specified
Don/Doff Information	No assistance necessary
Use/Reuse	Durable enough to be worn many times
Launderability	Not specified
Accessories	None

Special Requirements

Training Requirements	None
Training Available	None required
Manuals Available	None required
Surveillance Testing Requirements	Visual inspection before and after each use
Support Equipment	None
Testing Information	None required
Applicable Regulations	Not specified
Health Hazards	None
Communications Interface Capability	Not specified
EOD Compatibility	Not specified

General

Name	*Butyl Plus—NBC/Toxic Protective Glove*
Item # 9	
	Picture Not Available
Technology	Impermeable butyl/neoprene
Stock Number	NATO# 8415-99-130-9429 to 9434; Mfg# 39113-39116
Protection Type	Skin protection from Military CB Agents, ketones and esters; also resists oil/petroleum products
Equipment Category	Five finger protective glove with gauntlet
Availability	Full production. Delivery: 30 d to 60 d after order.
Current User(s)	Full commercial use and NATO and U.S. military use
Manufacturer	COMESEC Safety Inc.
Manufacturer Type	Private, Foreign/USA
Developer	COMESEC Safety Inc.
Source	Sales: INDEF Services Intl 14847 Lee Highway Amissville, VA 20106-0089 540-937-7327 (Tel) 540-937-7328 (Fax) indefsteve@msn.com
Certification	Meets OSHA PPE and NATO Military Standard

Operational Parameters

Chemical Warfare (CW) Agents Protected Against	All Military CW agents
Biological Warfare (BW) Agents Protected Against	All Military BW agents
Toxic Industrial (TIMs) Protected Against	Wide range of toxics including: ketones, acetates, ethylenes, and esters
Duration of Protection	Minimum 8 h against NATO standard challenge
Recommended Use(s)	Tactical operations, CBW response teams, and decontamination teams. Used with CB protective ensembles by ground personnel, air crews, and vehicle operators.

Physical Parameters

Sizes Available	S, M, L, and XL
Weight	10 oz (approximately)
Package Size and Volume	16 in x 5 in x 1 in—0.07 cuff
Power Requirements	None
Material Type	Impermeable butyl/neoprene rubber
Construction Type	Solvent dipped
Color	Available: black

Logistical Parameters

Ease of Use	Simple pull on—no training required
Consumables	None
Maintenance Requirements	None
Shelf Life	Estimated 4 yr to 5 yr
Transportability	Not applicable
Operational Limitations	Not for use near open flame
Environmental Conditions	0 °F to +140 °F. Maintains protection if wet.
Unit Cost	$26/pair
Maintenance Cost	None
Warranty	Replacement if manufacturing flaw found upon initial use within 12 mo of purchase
Don/Doff Information	Glove is worn over skin. Can don without assistance.
Use/Reuse	Use estimated 14 d in normal wear. Can be decontaminated.
Launderability	Able to be reused when decontaminated
Accessories	None

Special Requirements

Training Requirements	None
Training Available	None required
Manuals Available	None required
Surveillance Testing Requirements	Recommend periodic test of sample from each lot after 24 mo to 36 mo
Support Equipment	None
Testing Information	Meets NATO Standard Test Requirement for CB ensemble
Applicable Regulations	NATO/UK Spec. SC/4985B, MIL G–12223J and OSHA PPE Std.
Health Hazards	None
Communications Interface Capability	Not applicable
EOD Compatibility	Yes

General

Name	*Multi Plus—HazMat/Toxic Protective Glove*
Item # 10	
	Picture Not Available
Technology	Impermeable PVC/nitrile coated, interlock knit lining
Stock Number	Mfg #32443–32446 14 in length, #32663–32666 16 in length
Protection Type	Skin protection from HazMat/toxics also resists oil/petroleum products
Equipment Category	HazMat/toxic five-finger protective glove with gauntlet. Good wet/dry grip and perfect fit
Availability	Full production delivery: 30 d to 60 d after order
Current User(s)	Full commercial use
Manufacturer	COMESEC Safety Inc.
Manufacturer Type	Private, Foreign/USA
Developer	COMESEC Safety Inc.
Source	Sales: INDEF Services Intl. 14847 Lee Highway Amissville, VA 20106–0089 540–937–7327 (Tel) 540–937–7328 (Fax) indefsteve@msn.com
Certification	Meets OSHA PPE

Operational Parameters

Chemical Warfare (CW) Agents Protected Against	Not tested
Biological Warfare (BW) Agents Protected Against	Not tested
Toxic Industrial (TIMs) Protected Against	Protects against multiple TIMs. Wide range of toxics including: acids, oils, petroleum, and solvents.
Duration of Protection	Minimum 8 h in presence of toxics. Recommend use with under glove if direct handling required.
Recommended Use(s)	HazMat response teams, HazMat decontamination teams

Physical Parameters

Sizes Available	14 in length and 16 in length available—S, M, L, and XL
Weight	10 oz (approximately)
Package Size and Volume	16 in x 5 in x 1 in—0.07 cuff
Power Requirements	None
Material Type	Impermeable PVC/nitrile coated, interlock knit lining
Construction Type	Not specified
Color	Blue

Logistical Parameters

Ease of Use	Simple pull on - no training required
Consumables	None
Maintenance Requirements	None
Shelf Life	Estimated 3 yr to 5 yr
Transportability	Not applicable
Operational Limitations	Not for use near open flame
Environmental Conditions	-20 °F to +140 °F. Maintains protection if wet.
Unit Cost	$5/pair to $7.50/pair
Maintenance Cost	None
Warranty	Replacement if manufacturing flaw found upon initial use within 12 mo of purchase
Don/Doff Information	Glove is worn over skin. Can don without assistance. Can be worn with Silvershield (manufactured by North for extra protection if direct handling of HazMats required).
Use/Reuse	Recommend disposal after contamination
Launderability	Able to be cleaned and reused
Accessories	None

Special Requirements

Training Requirements	None
Training Available	None required
Manuals Available	None required
Surveillance Testing Requirements	Recommend periodic test of sample from each lot after 36 mo
Support Equipment	None
Testing Information	Meets OSHA PPE Standards
Applicable Regulations	OSHA, PPE Std.
Health Hazards	None
Communications Interface Capability	Not applicable
EOD Compatibility	Yes

General

Name — *Chemical Biological Protective Sock*
Item # 11

Picture Not Available

Technology	Permeable filter layer (CB filter material) with integrated outer face polyamide fabric and inner polyamide/cotton, all bonded in laminate
Stock Number	CBPS01—(standard sock)
Protection Type	Skin protection from Military Chemical/Biological Warfare Agents
Equipment Category	Protective sock, pull on with high comfort
Availability	Full Production anticipated by July 2000 Delivery: Standard Med – 60 d after order
Current User(s)	Versions in service with U.S. Navy, NATO Armed Forces, Civil Defense, and Malaysian Army
Manufacturer	CA Fashion Inc.
Manufacturer Type	Private, USA/Foreign
Developer	CEB
Source	Sales: INDEF Services Intl. 14847 Lee Highway Amissville, VA 20106–0089 540–937–7327 (Tel) 540–937–7328 (Fax) indefsteve@msn.com
Certification	Meets NATO Military Standard and tested to ERDEC Mil-Std by Natick

Operational Parameters

Chemical Warfare (CW) Agents Protected Against	All Military CW agents
Biological Warfare (BW) Agents Protected Against	All Military BW agents
Toxic Industrial (TIMs) Protected Against	Not applicable
Duration of Protection	Minimum 8 h against NATO standard challenge
Recommended Use(s)	Tactical operations, CBW response teams: Used with CB Protective Ensemble by ground personnel, air crews, and vehicle operators. Designed to be worn under boot.

Physical Parameters

Sizes Available	S, M, L, and XL
Weight	14 oz
Package Size and Volume	16 in x 6 in x 1.5 in—under 0.1 cuff
Power Requirements	None
Material Type	Permeable polyamide fabric face with integrated CB filter material and inner poly/cotton all bonded in laminate
Construction Type	Sewn
Color	Black

Logistical Parameters

Ease of Use	Simple pull on; no training required. Socks provide maximum comfort (even in hot/humid conditions).
Consumables	None
Maintenance Requirements	None
Shelf Life	Estimated 6 yr to 8 yr
Transportability	Not applicable
Operational Limitations	Not for use with industrial HazMat
Environmental Conditions	-30 °F to +140 °F. Maintains protection if wet.
Unit Cost	$27/pair
Maintenance Cost	None
Warranty	Replacement if manufacturing flaw found upon initial use within 12 mo of purchase
Don/Doff Information	Glove is worn over skin under boot. Can don without assistance.
Use/Reuse	Use minimum 14 d in normal wear
Launderability	Hand wash only up to 3 times (inspect for tears/wear after each)
Accessories	None

Special Requirements

Training Requirements	None
Training Available	None required
Manuals Available	None required
Surveillance Testing Requirements	Recommend periodic test of sample from each lot after 24 mo to 36 mo
Support Equipment	None
Testing Information	Meets NATO Standard Test Requirement for CB ensemble
Applicable Regulations	Not applicable
Health Hazards	None
Communications Interface Capability	Not applicable
EOD Compatibility	Yes

General

Name — Tyvek® Labcoat
Item # 12

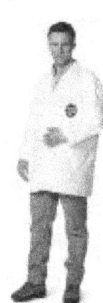

Technology	High density spunbonded polyethylene coated with polyethylene film
Stock Number	14300
Protection Type	Percutaneous
Equipment Category	Labcoat, snap front
Availability	Commercial
Current User(s)	U.S. Government/military, local government/fire department, emergency response teams, general industry, remediation companies, and chemical manufacturing. Specific organizations currently using item available upon request.
Manufacturer	DuPont Tyvek® Protective Apparel U.S. Highway #1 North McBee, SC 29101 800–845–6962 (Tel) 843–335–8599 (Fax) e-mail: Mary-Ann.Daniel@usa.dupont.com POC: M. A. Daniel 888–577–6960 (Tel)
Manufacturer Type	Domestic manufacturer
Developer	DuPont Protective Apparel
Source	DuPont Tyvek® Protective Apparel
Certification	Not applicable

Operational Parameters

Chemical Warfare (CW) Agents Protected Against	Not applicable
Biological Warfare (BW) Agents Protected Against	Not specified
Toxic Industrial (TIMs) Protected Against	Hazardous dry particulates. For specific test data, call the DuPont Protective Apparel Fax-on-Demand Service at 800–558–9329 and request document 610, or go to http://www.dupont.com/tyvek/protective-apparel htm.
Duration of Protection	For specific test data on hazardous dry particulates, call the DuPont Protective Apparel Fax-on-Demand Service at 800–558–9329 and request document 610, or go to http://www.dupont.com/tyvek/protective-apparel htm. No test data for CW agents.

Recommended Use(s)	Crisis management (post decontamination); remediation

Physical Parameters

Sizes Available	S through XXXXL. Additional sizes available upon request.
Weight	5 lb/container, 30 unit/container
Package Size and Volume	14 7/8 in L x 10 1/2 in W x 7 1/2 in H
Power Requirements	Not applicable
Material Type	High density spunbonded polyethylene coated with polyethylene film
Construction Type	Sewn seam—overedge serged seam construction offers protection against many dry particulates and light sprays
Color	White

Logistical Parameters

Ease of Use	Ergonomically designed for maximum mobility and flexibility
Consumables	None
Maintenance Requirements	Visual inspection prior to use
Shelf Life	Store in a cool, dry environment in original packaging. Manufacturer recommends designating "for training use only" after 5 yr of storage.
Transportability	Easily transported
Operational Limitations	Directly relates to the physical condition of user
Environmental Conditions	Can be used in all common outdoor weather conditions and climates. Rain, snow, extreme temperatures and humidity will have no effect on the suit.
Unit Cost	$101/carton
Maintenance Cost	Minimum labor cost for routine suit inspection
Warranty	90 d for workmanship and materials
Don/Doff Information	No assistance required for donning and doffing. Average donning and doffing time is minimal.
Use/Reuse	Discard after use. Decontamination specific to chemical exposure. Disposal per jurisdictional regulations. Can be incinerated provided garment is not contaminated with hazardous or toxic materials.
Launderability	Not applicable. Not intended for reuse after exposure to hazardous materials.
Accessories	None

Special Requirements

Training Requirements	No special training required
Training Available	Yes. DuPont will provide specialized group training upon request.
Manuals Available	None required
Surveillance Testing Requirements	Visual inspection (for holes and tears) prior to use

Support Equipment	Appropriate respiratory, foot, eye/face, hand, and head protection
Testing Information	Physical properties: Basis weight (ASTM D3776–85) 1.2 oz/yd^2 Thickness (ASTM D1777–64) 5.3 mils Strip tensile (in-lb) (ASTM D1682)(MD/CD) 7.9/7.6 Work to break (in-lb) (ASTM D1682) (MD/CD) 2.4/2.1 Tongue tear, lb (ASTM D2261 (MD/CD) Barrier data available by calling 877–797–5907 or go to http://www.dupont.com/tyvek/protective-apparel.htm.
Applicable Regulations	None
Health Hazards	None
Communications Interface Capability	Not applicable
EOD Compatibility	Compatible with EOD suit

General

Name *Tyvek® Labcoat*

Item # 13

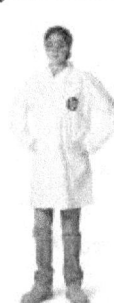

Technology	High density spunbonded polyethylene coated with polyethylene film
Stock Number	14301
Protection Type	Percutaneous
Equipment Category	Labcoat, snap front, and 2 pockets
Availability	Commercial
Current User(s)	U.S. Government/military, local government/fire department, emergency response teams, general industry, remediation companies, and chemical manufacturing. Specific organizations currently using item available upon request.
Manufacturer	DuPont Tyvek® Protective Apparel U.S. Highway #1 North McBee, SC 29101 800–845–6962 (Tel) 843–335–8599 (Fax) e-mail: Mary-Ann.Daniel@usa.dupont.com POC: M. A. Daniel 888–577–6960 (Tel)
Manufacturer Type	Domestic manufacturer
Developer	DuPont Protective Apparel
Source	DuPont Tyvek® Protective Apparel
Certification	Not applicable

Operational Parameters

Chemical Warfare (CW) Agents Protected Against	Not applicable
Biological Warfare (BW) Agents Protected Against	Not specified
Toxic Industrial (TIMs) Protected Against	Hazardous dry particulates. For specific test data, call the DuPont Protective Apparel Fax-on-Demand Service at 800–558–9329 and request document 610, or go to http://www.dupont.com/tyvek/protective-apparel htm.
Duration of Protection	For specific test data on hazardous dry particulates, call the DuPont Protective Apparel Fax-on-Demand Service at 800–558–9329 and request document 610, or go to http://www.dupont.com/tyvek/protective-apparel.htm. No test data for CW agents.
Recommended Use(s)	Crisis management (post decontamination); remediation

Physical Parameters

Sizes Available	S through XXXXL. Additional sizes available upon request.
Weight	5 lb/container, 30 unit/container
Package Size and Volume	14 7/8 in L x 10 1/2 in W x 7 1/2 in H
Power Requirements	Not applicable
Material Type	High density spunbonded polyethylene coated with polyethylene film
Construction Type	Sewn seam—overedge serged seam construction offers protection against many dry particulates and light sprays
Color	White

Logistical Parameters

Ease of Use	Ergonomically designed for maximum mobility and flexibility
Consumables	None
Maintenance Requirements	Visual inspection prior to use
Shelf Life	Store in a cool, dry environment in original packaging. Manufacturer recommends designating "for training use only" after 5 yr of storage.
Transportability	Easily transported
Operational Limitations	Directly relates to the physical condition of user
Environmental Conditions	Can be used in all common outdoor weather conditions and climates. Rain, snow, extreme temperatures and humidity will have no effect on the suit.
Unit Cost	$102/carton
Maintenance Cost	Minimum labor cost for routine suit inspection
Warranty	90 d for workmanship and materials
Don/Doff Information	No assistance required for donning and doffing. Average donning and doffing time is minimal.
Use/Reuse	Discard after use. Decontamination specific to chemical exposure. Disposal per jurisdictional regulations. Can be incinerated provided garment is not contaminated with hazardous or toxic materials.
Launderability	Not applicable. Not intended for reuse after exposure to hazardous materials.
Accessories	None

Special Requirements

Training Requirements	No special training required
Training Available	Yes. DuPont will provide specialized group training upon request.
Manuals Available	None required
Surveillance Testing Requirements	Visual inspection (for holes and tears) prior to use
Support Equipment	Appropriate respiratory, foot, eye/face, hand, and head protection

Testing Information	Physical properties: Basis weight (ASTM D3776–85) 1.2 oz/yd^2 Thickness (ASTM D1777–64) 5.3 mils Strip tensile (in-lb) (ASTM D1682)(MD/CD) 7.9/7.6 Work to break (in-lb) (ASTM D1682) (MD/CD) 2.4/2.1 Tongue tear, lb (ASTM D2261 (MD/CD) Barrier data available by calling 877–797–5907 or go to http://www.dupont.com/tyvek/protective-apparel.htm.
Applicable Regulations	None
Health Hazards	None
Communications Interface Capability	Not applicable
EOD Compatibility	Compatible with EOD suit

General

Name   *Tyvek® Shirt*
Item # 14

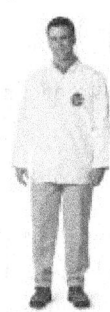

Technology	High density spunbonded polyethylene coated with polyethylene film
Stock Number	14303
Protection Type	Percutaneous
Equipment Category	Shirt, snap front, and long sleeves
Availability	Commercial
Current User(s)	U.S. Government/military, local government/fire department, emergency response teams, general industry, remediation companies, and chemical manufacturing. Specific organizations currently using item available upon request.
Manufacturer	DuPont Tyvek® Protective Apparel U.S. Highway #1 North McBee, SC 29101 800–845–6962 (Tel) 843–335–8599 (Fax) e-mail: Mary-Ann.Daniel@usa.dupont.com POC: M. A. Daniel 888–577–6960 (Tel)
Manufacturer Type	Domestic manufacturer
Developer	DuPont Protective Apparel
Source	DuPont Tyvek® Protective Apparel
Certification	Not applicable

Operational Parameters

Chemical Warfare (CW) Agents Protected Against	Not applicable
Biological Warfare (BW) Agents Protected Against	Not specified
Toxic Industrial (TIMs) Protected Against	Hazardous dry particulates. For specific test data, call the DuPont Protective Apparel Fax-on-Demand Service at 800–558–9329 and request document 610, or go to http://www.dupont.com/tyvek/protective-apparel.htm.
Duration of Protection	For specific test data on hazardous dry particulates, call the DuPont Protective Apparel Fax-on-Demand Service at 800–558–9329 and request document 610, or go to http://www.dupont.com/tyvek/protective-apparel.htm. No test data for CW agents.

Recommended Use(s)	Crisis management (post decontamination); remediation
Physical Parameters	
Sizes Available	S through XXXXL. Additional sizes available upon request.
Weight	5 lb/container, 30 unit/container
Package Size and Volume	14 7/8 in L x 10 1/2 in W x 7 1/2 in H
Power Requirements	Not applicable
Material Type	High density spunbonded polyethylene coated with polyethylene film
Construction Type	Sewn seam—overedge serged seam construction offers protection against many dry particulates and light sprays
Color	White
Logistical Parameters	
Ease of Use	Ergonomically designed for maximum mobility and flexibility
Consumables	None
Maintenance Requirements	Visual inspection prior to use
Shelf Life	Store in a cool, dry environment in original packaging. Manufacturer recommends designating "for training use only" after 5 yr of storage.
Transportability	Easily transported
Operational Limitations	Directly relates to the physical condition of user
Environmental Conditions	Can be used in all common outdoor weather conditions and climates. Rain, snow, extreme temperatures and humidity will have no effect on the suit.
Unit Cost	$98/carton
Maintenance Cost	Minimum labor cost for routine suit inspection
Warranty	90 d for workmanship and materials
Don/Doff Information	No assistance required for donning and doffing. Average donning and doffing time is minimal.
Use/Reuse	Discard after use. Decontamination specific to chemical exposure. Disposal per jurisdictional regulations. Can be incinerated provided garment is not contaminated with hazardous or toxic materials.
Launderability	Not applicable. Not intended for reuse after exposure to hazardous materials.
Accessories	None
Special Requirements	
Training Requirements	No special training required
Training Available	Yes. DuPont will provide specialized group training upon request.
Manuals Available	None required
Surveillance Testing Requirements	Visual inspection (for holes and tears) prior to use

Support Equipment	Appropriate respiratory, foot, eye/face, hand, and head protection
Testing Information	Physical properties: Basis weight (ASTM D3776–85) 1.2 oz/yd^2 Thickness (ASTM D1777–64) 5.3 mils Strip tensile (in-lb) (ASTM D1682)(MD/CD) 7.9/7.6 Work to break (in-lb) (ASTM D1682) (MD/CD) 2.4/2.1 Tongue tear, lb (ASTM D2261 (MD/CD) Barrier data available by calling 877–797–5907 or go to http://www.dupont.com/tyvek/protective-apparel htm.
Applicable Regulations	None
Health Hazards	None
Communications Interface Capability	Not applicable
EOD Compatibility	Compatible with EOD suit

General

Name — Tyvek® Labcoat
Item # 15

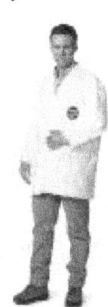

Technology	High density spunbonded polyethylene coated with polyethylene film. Pictured is stock # 14300
Stock Number	14344
Protection Type	Percutaneous
Equipment Category	Labcoat, snap front, 2 pockets, and elastic wrist
Availability	Commercial
Current User(s)	U.S. Government/military, local government/fire department, emergency response teams, general industry, remediation companies, and chemical manufacturing. Specific organizations currently using item available upon request.
Manufacturer	DuPont Tyvek® Protective Apparel U.S. Highway #1 North McBee, SC 29101 800–845–6962 (Tel) 843–335–8599 (Fax) e-mail: Mary-Ann.Daniel@usa.dupont.com POC: M. A. Daniel 888–577–6960 (Tel)
Manufacturer Type	Domestic manufacturer
Developer	DuPont Protective Apparel
Source	DuPont Tyvek® Protective Apparel
Certification	Not applicable

Operational Parameters

Chemical Warfare (CW) Agents Protected Against	Not applicable
Biological Warfare (BW) Agents Protected Against	Not specified
Toxic Industrial (TIMs) Protected Against	Hazardous dry particulates. For specific test data, call the DuPont Protective Apparel Fax-on-Demand Service at 800–558–9329 and request document 610, or go to http://www.dupont.com/tyvek/protective-apparel.htm.
Duration of Protection	For specific test data on hazardous dry particulates, call the DuPont Protective Apparel Fax-on-Demand Service at 800–558–9329 and request document 610, or go to http://www.dupont.com/tyvek/protective-apparel.htm. No test data for CW agents.
Recommended Use(s)	Crisis management (post decontamination); remediation

Physical Parameters

Sizes Available	S through XXXXL. Additional sizes available upon request.
Weight	6 lb/container, 30 unit/container
Package Size and Volume	14 7/8 in L x 10 1/2 in W x 7 1/2 in H
Power Requirements	Not applicable
Material Type	High density spunbonded polyethylene coated with polyethylene film
Construction Type	Sewn sea—overedge serged seam construction offers protection against many dry particulates and light sprays
Color	White

Logistical Parameters

Ease of Use	Ergonomically designed for maximum mobility and flexibility
Consumables	None
Maintenance Requirements	Visual inspection prior to use
Shelf Life	Store in a cool, dry environment in original packaging. Manufacturer recommends designating "for training use only" after 5 yr of storage.
Transportability	Easily transported
Operational Limitations	Directly relates to the physical condition of user
Environmental Conditions	Can be used in all common outdoor weather conditions and climates. Rain, snow, extreme temperatures and humidity will have no effect on the suit.
Unit Cost	$123/carton
Maintenance Cost	Minimum labor cost for routine suit inspection
Warranty	90 d for workmanship and materials
Don/Doff Information	No assistance required for donning and doffing. Average donning and doffing time is minimal.
Use/Reuse	Discard after use. Decontamination specific to chemical exposure. Disposal per jurisdictional regulations. Can be incinerated provided garment is not contaminated with hazardous or toxic materials.
Launderability	Not applicable. Not intended for reuse after exposure to hazardous materials.
Accessories	None

Special Requirements

Training Requirements	No special training required
Training Available	Yes. DuPont will provide specialized group training upon request.
Manuals Available	None required
Surveillance Testing Requirements	Visual inspection (for holes and tears) prior to use
Support Equipment	Appropriate respiratory, foot, eye/face, hand, and head protection

Testing Information	Physical properties: Basis weight (ASTM D3776–85) 1.2 oz/yd^2 Thickness (ASTM D1777–64) 5.3 mils Strip tensile (in-lb) (ASTM D1682)(MD/CD) 7.9/7.6 Work to break (in-lb) (ASTM D1682) (MD/CD) 2.4/2.1 Tongue tear, lb (ASTM D2261 (MD/CD) Barrier data available by calling 877–797–5907 or go to http://www.dupont.com/tyvek/protective-apparel.htm.
Applicable Regulations	None
Health Hazards	None
Communications Interface Capability	Not applicable
EOD Compatibility	Compatible with EOD suit

General

Name	*Tyvek® Labcoat*
Item # 16	

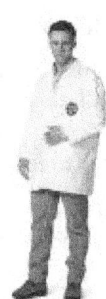

Technology	High density spunbonded polyethylene coated with polyethylene film Pictured is stock # 14300
Stock Number	14347
Protection Type	Percutaneous
Equipment Category	Labcoat, snap front, and elastic wrist
Availability	Commercial
Current User(s)	U.S. Government/military, local government/fire department, emergency response teams, general industry, remediation companies, and chemical manufacturing. Specific organizations currently using item available upon request.
Manufacturer	DuPont Tyvek® Protective Apparel U.S. Highway #1 North McBee, SC 29101 800–845–6962 (Tel) 843–335–8599 (Fax) e-mail: Mary-Ann.Daniel@usa.dupont.com POC: M. A. Daniel 888–577–6960 (Tel)
Manufacturer Type	Domestic manufacturer
Developer	DuPont Protective Apparel
Source	DuPont Tyvek® Protective Apparel
Certification	Not applicable

Operational Parameters

Chemical Warfare (CW) Agents Protected Against	Not applicable
Biological Warfare (BW) Agents Protected Against	Not specified
Toxic Industrial (TIMs) Protected Against	Hazardous dry particulates. For specific test data, call the DuPont Protective Apparel Fax-on-Demand Service at 800–558–9329 and request document 610, or go to http://www.dupont.com/tyvek/protective-apparel.htm.
Duration of Protection	For specific test data on hazardous dry particulates, call the DuPont Protective Apparel Fax-on-Demand Service at 800–558–9329 and request document 610, or go to http://www.dupont.com/tyvek/protective-apparel.htm. No test data for CW agents.
Recommended Use(s)	Crisis management (post decontamination); remediation

Physical Parameters

Sizes Available	S through XXXXL. Additional sizes available upon request.
Weight	6 lb/container, 30 unit/container
Package Size and Volume	14 7/8 in L x 10 1/2 in W x 7 1/2 in H
Power Requirements	Not applicable
Material Type	High density spunbonded polyethylene coated with polyethylene film
Construction Type	Sewn seam—overedge serged seam construction offers protection against many dry particulates and light sprays
Color	White

Logistical Parameters

Ease of Use	Ergonomically designed for maximum mobility and flexibility
Consumables	None
Maintenance Requirements	Visual inspection prior to use
Shelf Life	Store in a cool, dry environment in original packaging. Manufacturer recommends designating "for training use only" after 5 yr of storage.
Transportability	Easily transported
Operational Limitations	Directly relates to the physical condition of user
Environmental Conditions	Can be used in all common outdoor weather conditions and climates. Rain, snow, extreme temperatures and humidity will have no effect on the suit.
Unit Cost	$112/carton
Maintenance Cost	Minimum labor cost for routine suit inspection
Warranty	90 d for workmanship and materials
Don/Doff Information	No assistance required for donning and doffing. Average donning and doffing time is minimal.
Use/Reuse	Discard after use. Decontamination specific to chemical exposure. Disposal per jurisdictional regulations. Can be incinerated provided garment is not contaminated with hazardous or toxic materials.
Launderability	Not applicable. Not intended for reuse after exposure to hazardous materials.
Accessories	None

Special Requirements

Training Requirements	No special training required
Training Available	Yes. DuPont will provide specialized group training upon request.
Manuals Available	None required
Surveillance Testing Requirements	Visual inspection (for holes and tears) prior to use
Support Equipment	Appropriate respiratory, foot, eye/face, hand, and head protection

Testing Information	Physical properties: Basis weight (ASTM D3776–85) 1.2 oz/yd^2 Thickness (ASTM D1777–64) 5.3 mils Strip tensile (in-lb) (ASTM D1682)(MD/CD) 7.9/7.6 Work to break (in-lb) (ASTM D1682) (MD/CD) 2.4/2.1 Tongue tear, lb (ASTM D2261 (MD/CD) Barrier data available by calling 877–797–5907 or go to http://www.dupont.com/tyvek/protective-apparel htm.
Applicable Regulations	None
Health Hazards	None
Communications Interface Capability	Not applicable
EOD Compatibility	Compatible with EOD suit

General

Name *Tyvek® Pants*

Item # 17

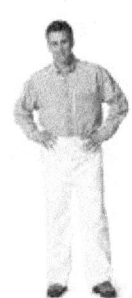

Technology	High density spunbonded polyethylene coated with polyethylene film
Stock Number	14350
Protection Type	Percutaneous
Equipment Category	Pants, elastic waist
Availability	Commercial
Current User(s)	U.S. Government/military, local government/fire department, emergency response teams, general industry, remediation companies, and chemical manufacturing. Specific organizations currently using item available upon request.
Manufacturer	DuPont Tyvek® Protective Apparel U.S. Highway #1 North McBee, SC 29101 800–845–6962 (Tel) 843–335–8599 (Fax) e-mail: Mary-Ann.Daniel@usa.dupont.com POC: M. A. Daniel 888–577–6960 (Tel)
Manufacturer Type	Domestic manufacturer
Developer	DuPont Protective Apparel
Source	DuPont Tyvek® Protective Apparel
Certification	Not applicable

Operational Parameters

Chemical Warfare (CW) Agents Protected Against	Not applicable
Biological Warfare (BW) Agents Protected Against	Not specified
Toxic Industrial (TIMs) Protected Against	Hazardous dry particulates. For specific test data, call the DuPont Protective Apparel Fax-on-Demand Service at 800–558–9329 and request document 610, or go to http://www.dupont.com/tyvek/protective-apparel htm.
Duration of Protection	For specific test data on hazardous dry particulates, call the DuPont Protective Apparel Fax-on-Demand Service at 800–558–9329 and request document 610, or go to http://www.dupont.com/tyvek/protective-apparel htm. No test data for CW agents.

Recommended Use(s)	Crisis management (post decontamination); remediation
Physical Parameters	
Sizes Available	S through XXXXL. Additional sizes available upon request.
Weight	5 lb/container, 30 unit/container
Package Size and Volume	14 7/8 in L x 10 1/2 in W x 7 1/2 in H
Power Requirements	Not applicable
Material Type	High density spunbonded polyethylene coated with polyethylene film
Construction Type	Sewn seam—overedge serged seam construction offers protection against many dry particulates and light sprays
Color	White
Logistical Parameters	
Ease of Use	Ergonomically designed for maximum mobility and flexibility
Consumables	None
Maintenance Requirements	Visual inspection prior to use
Shelf Life	Store in a cool, dry environment in original packaging. Manufacturer recommends designating "for training use only" after 5 yr of storage.
Transportability	Easily transported
Operational Limitations	Directly relates to the physical condition of user
Environmental Conditions	Can be used in all common outdoor weather conditions and climates. Rain, snow, extreme temperatures and humidity will have no effect on the suit.
Unit Cost	$79/carton
Maintenance Cost	Minimum labor cost for routine suit inspection
Warranty	90 d for workmanship and materials
Don/Doff Information	No assistance required for donning and doffing. Average donning and doffing time is minimal.
Use/Reuse	Discard after use. Decontamination specific to chemical exposure. Disposal per jurisdictional regulations. Can be incinerated provided garment is not contaminated with hazardous or toxic materials.
Launderability	Not applicable. Not intended for reuse after exposure to hazardous materials.
Accessories	None
Special Requirements	
Training Requirements	No special training required
Training Available	Yes. DuPont will provide specialized group training upon request.
Manuals Available	None required
Surveillance Testing Requirements	Visual inspection (for holes and tears) prior to use

Support Equipment	Appropriate respiratory, foot, eye/face, hand, and head protection
Testing Information	Physical properties: Basis weight (ASTM D3776–85) 1.2 oz/yd^2 Thickness (ASTM D1777–64) 5.3 mils Strip tensile (in-lb) (ASTM D1682)(MD/CD) 7.9/7.6 Work to break (in-lb) (ASTM D1682) (MD/CD) 2.4/2.1 Tongue tear, lb (ASTM D2261 (MD/CD) Barrier data available by calling 877–797–5907 or go to http://www.dupont.com/tyvek/protective-apparel htm.
Applicable Regulations	None
Health Hazards	None
Communications Interface Capability	Not applicable
EOD Compatibility	Compatible with EOD suit

General

Name — *Tyvek® Hood*
Item # 18

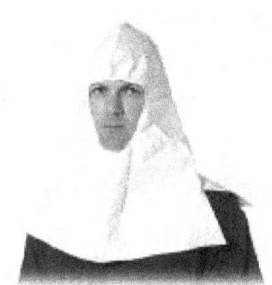

Technology	High density spunbonded polyethylene coated with polyethylene film
Stock Number	14383
Protection Type	Percutaneous
Equipment Category	Hood, pull over, chest length, and elastic face
Availability	Commercial
Current User(s)	U.S. Government/military, local government/fire department, emergency response teams, general industry, remediation companies, and chemical manufacturing. Specific organizations currently using item available upon request.
Manufacturer	DuPont Tyvek® Protective Apparel U.S. Highway #1 North McBee, SC 29101 800–845–6962 (Tel) 843–335–8599 (Fax) e-mail: Mary-Ann.Daniel@usa.dupont.com POC: M. A. Daniel 888–577–6960 (Tel)
Manufacturer Type	Domestic manufacturer
Developer	DuPont Protective Apparel
Source	DuPont Tyvek® Protective Apparel
Certification	Not applicable

Operational Parameters

Chemical Warfare (CW) Agents Protected Against	Not applicable
Biological Warfare (BW) Agents Protected Against	Not specified
Toxic Industrial (TIMs) Protected Against	Hazardous dry particulates. For specific test data, call the DuPont Protective Apparel Fax-on-Demand Service at 800–558–9329 and request document 610, or go to http://www.dupont.com/tyvek/protective-apparel.htm.
Duration of Protection	For specific test data on hazardous dry particulates, call the DuPont Protective Apparel Fax-on-Demand Service at 800–558–9329 and request document 610, or go to http://www.dupont.com/tyvek/protective-apparel.htm. No test data for CW agents.

Recommended Use(s)	Crisis management (post decontamination); remediation

Physical Parameters

Sizes Available	S through XXXXL. Additional sizes available upon request.
Weight	4 lb/container, 100 unit/container
Package Size and Volume	14 7/8 in L x 10 1/2 in W x 7 1/2 in H
Power Requirements	Not applicable
Material Type	High density spunbonded polyethylene coated with polyethylene film
Construction Type	Sewn seam—overedge serged seam construction offers protection against many dry particulates and light sprays
Color	White

Logistical Parameters

Ease of Use	Ergonomically designed for maximum mobility and flexibility
Consumables	None
Maintenance Requirements	Visual inspection prior to use
Shelf Life	Store in a cool, dry environment in original packaging. Manufacturer recommends designating "for training use only" after 5 yr of storage.
Transportability	Easily transported
Operational Limitations	Directly relates to the physical condition of user
Environmental Conditions	Can be used in all common outdoor weather conditions and climates. Rain, snow, extreme temperatures and humidity will have no effect on the suit.
Unit Cost	$114/carton
Maintenance Cost	Minimum labor cost for routine suit inspection
Warranty	90 d for workmanship and materials
Don/Doff Information	No assistance required for donning and doffing. Average donning and doffing time is minimal.
Use/Reuse	Discard after use. Decontamination specific to chemical exposure. Disposal per jurisdictional regulations. Can be incinerated provided garment is not contaminated with hazardous or toxic materials.
Launderability	Not applicable. Not intended for reuse after exposure to hazardous materials.
Accessories	None

Special Requirements

Training Requirements	No special training required
Training Available	Yes. DuPont will provide specialized group training upon request.
Manuals Available	None required
Surveillance Testing Requirements	Visual inspection (for holes and tears) prior to use

Support Equipment	Appropriate respiratory, foot, hand, and head protection
Testing Information	Physical properties: Basis weight (ASTM D3776–85) 1.2 oz/yd^2 Thickness (ASTM D1777–64) 5.3 mils Strip tensile (in-lb) (ASTM D1682)(MD/CD) 7.9/7.6 Work to break (in-lb) (ASTM D1682) (MD/CD) 2.4/2.1 Tongue tear, lb (ASTM D2261 (MD/CD) Barrier data available by calling 877–797–5907 or go to http://www.dupont.com/tyvek/protective-apparel htm.
Applicable Regulations	None
Health Hazards	None
Communications Interface Capability	Not applicable
EOD Compatibility	Compatible with EOD suit

General

Name — *Tyvek® Hood*
Item # 19

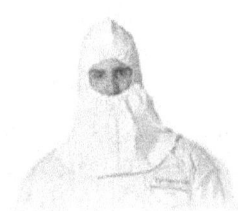

Technology	High density spunbonded polyethylene coated with polyethylene film
Stock Number	14386
Protection Type	Percutaneous
Equipment Category	Hood, pull over, shoulder length, and elastic face
Availability	Commercial
Current User(s)	U.S. Government/military, local government/fire department, emergency response teams, general industry, remediation companies, and chemical manufacturing. Specific organizations currently using item available upon request.
Manufacturer	DuPont Tyvek® Protective Apparel U.S. Highway #1 North McBee, SC 29101 800–845–6962 (Tel) 843–335–8599 (Fax) e-mail: Mary-Ann.Daniel@usa.dupont.com POC: M. A. Daniel 888–577–6960 (Tel)
Manufacturer Type	Domestic manufacturer
Developer	DuPont Protective Apparel
Source	DuPont Tyvek® Protective Apparel
Certification	Not applicable

Operational Parameters

Chemical Warfare (CW) Agents Protected Against	Not applicable
Biological Warfare (BW) Agents Protected Against	Not specified
Toxic Industrial (TIMs) Protected Against	Hazardous dry particulates. For specific test data, call the DuPont Protective Apparel Fax-on-Demand Service at 800–558–9329 and request document 610, or go to http://www.dupont.com/tyvek/protective-apparel htm.
Duration of Protection	For specific test data on hazardous dry particulates, call the DuPont Protective Apparel Fax-on-Demand Service at 800–558–9329 and request document 610, or go to http://www.dupont.com/tyvek/protective-apparel htm. No test data for CW agents.

Recommended Use(s)	Crisis management (post decontamination); remediation

Physical Parameters

Sizes Available	Sm through XXXXL. Additional sizes available upon request.
Weight	4 lb/container, 100 unit/container
Package Size and Volume	14 7/8 in L x 10 1/2 in W x 7 1/2 in H
Power Requirements	Not applicable
Material Type	High density spunbonded polyethylene coated with polyethylene film
Construction Type	Sewn seam—overedge serged seam construction offers protection against many dry particulates and light sprays
Color	White

Logistical Parameters

Ease of Use	Ergonomically designed for maximum mobility and flexibility
Consumables	None
Maintenance Requirements	Visual inspection prior to use
Shelf Life	Store in a cool, dry environment in original packaging. Manufacturer recommends designating "for training use only" after 5 yr of storage.
Transportability	Easily transported
Operational Limitations	Directly relates to the physical condition of user
Environmental Conditions	Can be used in all common outdoor weather conditions and climates. Rain, snow, extreme temperatures and humidity will have no effect on the suit.
Unit Cost	$100/carton
Maintenance Cost	Minimum labor cost for routine suit inspection
Warranty	90 d for workmanship and materials
Don/Doff Information	No assistance required for donning and doffing. Average donning and doffing time is minimal.
Use/Reuse	Discard after use. Decontamination specific to chemical exposure. Disposal per jurisdictional regulations. Can be incinerated provided garment is not contaminated with hazardous or toxic materials.
Launderability	Not applicable. Not intended for reuse after exposure to hazardous materials.
Accessories	None

Special Requirements

Training Requirements	No special training required
Training Available	Yes. DuPont will provide specialized group training upon request.
Manuals Available	None required
Surveillance Testing Requirements	Visual inspection (for holes and tears) prior to use

Support Equipment	Appropriate respiratory, foot, hand, and head protection
Testing Information	Physical properties: Basis weight (ASTM D3776–85) 1.2 oz/yd^2 Thickness (ASTM D1777–64) 5.3 mils Strip tensile (in-lb) (ASTM D1682)(MD/CD) 7.9/7.6 Work to break (in-lb) (ASTM D1682) (MD/CD) 2.4/2.1 Tongue tear, lb (ASTM D2261 (MD/CD) Barrier data available by calling 877–797–5907 or go to http://www.dupont.com/tyvek/protective-apparel.htm.
Applicable Regulations	None
Health Hazards	None
Communications Interface Capability	Not applicable
EOD Compatibility	Compatible with EOD suit

General

Name — *Tyvek® Hood*
Item # 20

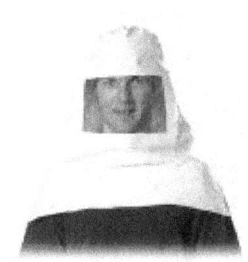

Technology	High density spunbonded polyethylene coated with polyethylene film
Stock Number	14388
Protection Type	Percutaneous
Equipment Category	Hood, pull over, shoulder length, and face shield
Availability	Commercial
Current User(s)	U.S. Government/military, local government/fire department, emergency response teams, general industry, remediation companies, and chemical manufacturing. Specific organizations currently using item available upon request.
Manufacturer	DuPont Tyvek® Protective Apparel U.S. Highway #1 North McBee, SC 29101 800–845–6962 (Tel) 843–335–8599 (Fax) e-mail: Mary-Ann.Daniel@usa.dupont.com POC: M. A. Daniel 888–577–6960 (Tel)
Manufacturer Type	Domestic manufacturer
Developer	DuPont Protective Apparel
Source	DuPont Tyvek® Protective Apparel
Certification	Not applicable

Operational Parameters

Chemical Warfare (CW) Agents Protected Against	Not applicable
Biological Warfare (BW) Agents Protected Against	Not specified
Toxic Industrial (TIMs) Protected Against	Hazardous dry particulates. For specific test data, call the DuPont Protective Apparel Fax-on-Demand Service at 800–558–9329 and request document 610, or go to http://www.dupont.com/tyvek/protective-apparel htm.
Duration of Protection	For specific test data on hazardous dry particulates, call the DuPont Protective Apparel Fax-on-Demand Service at 800–558–9329 and request document 610, or go to http://www.dupont.com/tyvek/protective-apparel htm. No test data for CW agents.

Recommended Use(s)	Crisis management (post decontamination); remediation

Physical Parameters

Sizes Available	S through XXXXL. Additional sizes available upon request.
Weight	3 lb/container, 25 unit/container
Package Size and Volume	14 7/8 in L x 10 1/2 in W x 7 1/2 in H
Power Requirements	Not applicable
Material Type	High density spunbonded polyethylene coated with polyethylene film
Construction Type	Sewn seam—overedge serged seam construction offers protection against many dry particulates and light sprays
Color	White

Logistical Parameters

Ease of Use	Ergonomically designed for maximum mobility and flexibility
Consumables	None
Maintenance Requirements	Visual inspection prior to use
Shelf Life	Store in a cool, dry environment in original packaging. Manufacturer recommends designating "for training use only" after five years storage.
Transportability	Easily transported
Operational Limitations	Directly relates to the physical condition of user
Environmental Conditions	Can be used in all common outdoor weather conditions and climates. Rain, snow, extreme temperatures and humidity will have no effect on the suit.
Unit Cost	$80/carton
Maintenance Cost	Minimum labor cost for routine suit inspection
Warranty	90 d for workmanship and materials
Don/Doff Information	No assistance required for donning and doffing. Average donning and doffing time is minimal.
Use/Reuse	Discard after use. Decontamination specific to chemical exposure. Disposal per jurisdictional regulations. Can be incinerated provided garment is not contaminated with hazardous or toxic materials.
Launderability	Not applicable. Not intended for reuse after exposure to hazardous materials.
Accessories	None

Special Requirements

Training Requirements	No special training required
Training Available	Yes. DuPont will provide specialized group training upon request.
Manuals Available	None required
Surveillance Testing Requirements	Visual inspection (for holes and tears) prior to use

Support Equipment	Appropriate respiratory, foot, hand, and head protection
Testing Information	Physical properties: Basis weight (ASTM D3776–85) 1.2 oz/yd^2 Thickness (ASTM D1777–64) 5.3 mils Strip tensile (in-lb) (ASTM D1682)(MD/CD) 7.9/7.6 Work to break (in-lb) (ASTM D1682) (MD/CD) 2.4/2.1 Tongue tear, lb (ASTM D2261 (MD/CD) Barrier data available by calling 877–797–5907 or go to http://www.dupont.com/tyvek/protective-apparel htm.
Applicable Regulations	None
Health Hazards	None
Communications Interface Capability	Not applicable
EOD Compatibility	Compatible with EOD suit

General

Name *Tychem® QC Labcoat*

Item # 21

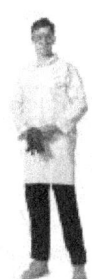

Technology	Selectively impermeable composite consisting of thermoplastic barrier films laminated to high strength thermoplastic nonwoven fabrics
Stock Number	35300
Protection Type	Percutaneous
Equipment Category	Labcoat, snap front
Availability	Commercial
Current User(s)	U.S. Government/military, local government/fire department, emergency response teams, general industry, remediation companies, and chemical manufacturing. Specific organizations currently using item available upon request.
Manufacturer	DuPont Tyvek® Protective Apparel U.S. Highway #1 North McBee, SC 29101 800–845–6962 (Tel) 843–335–8599 (Fax) e-mail: Mary-Ann.Daniel@usa.dupont.com POC: M. A. Daniel 888–577–6960 (Tel)
Manufacturer Type	Domestic manufacturer
Developer	DuPont Protective Apparel
Source	DuPont Tyvek® Protective Apparel
Certification	Not applicable

Operational Parameters

Chemical Warfare (CW) Agents Protected Against	Not tested
Biological Warfare (BW) Agents Protected Against	Not specified
Toxic Industrial (TIMs) Protected Against	Many inorganic acids, bases, and other liquid chemicals such as pesticides. For specific test data, call the DuPont Protective Apparel Fax-on-Demand Service at 800–558–9329 and request document 616, or go to http://www.dupont.com/tyvek/protective-apparel.htm.
Duration of Protection	For specific test data on TIMs, call the DuPont Protective Apparel Fax-on-Demand Service at 800–558–9329 and request document 616, or go to http://www.dupont.com/tyvek/protective-apparel.htm. No test data available for CW agents
Recommended Use(s)	Crisis management (post decontamination); medical triage; and remediation

Physical Parameters

Sizes Available	S through XXXXL. Additional sizes available upon request.
Weight	5 lb/container, 12 units/container
Package Size and Volume	14 7/8 in L x 10 in W x 10 in H
Power Requirements	Not applicable
Material Type	Selectively impermeable composite consisting of thermoplastic barrier films laminated to high strength thermoplastic nonwoven fabrics
Construction Type	Sewn seam—overedge serged seam construction offers protection against many dry particulates and light sprays
Color	Yellow, Grey

Logistical Parameters

Ease of Use	Ergonomically designed for maximum mobility and flexibility
Consumables	None
Maintenance Requirements	Visual inspection prior to use
Shelf Life	Store in a cool, dry environment in original packaging. Manufacturer recommends designating "for training use only" after 5 yr of storage.
Transportability	Easily transported
Operational Limitations	Directly relates to the physical condition of user
Environmental Conditions	Can be used in all common outdoor weather conditions and climates. Rain, snow, extreme temperatures and humidity will have no effect on the suit.
Unit Cost	$59/carton
Maintenance Cost	Minimum labor cost for routine suit inspection
Warranty	90 d for workmanship and materials
Don/Doff Information	No assistance required for donning and doffing. Average donning and doffing time is minimal.
Use/Reuse	Discard after use. Decontamination specific to chemical exposure. Disposal per jurisdictional regulations.
Launderability	Not applicable. Not intended for reuse after exposure to toxic chemicals. Dirt and dust can be manually removed with soap and water.
Accessories	None

Special Requirements

Training Requirements	No special training required
Training Available	Yes. DuPont will provide specialized group training upon request.
Manuals Available	Permeation Guide available
Surveillance Testing Requirements	Visual inspection (for holes and tears) prior to use
Support Equipment	Appropriate respiratory, foot, eye/face, hand, and head protection

Testing Information	Physical properties: Basis weight (ASTM D3776–85) 2.1 oz/yd^2 Thickness (ASTM D1777–64) 6.0 mils Mullen burst (ASTM D3786–87) 66 psi Breaking strength—Grab (md/xd) (ASTM D1682–64, sec. 5.3) 25/35 lb Tearing strength—Trapezoid (md/xd) (ASTM D1117–80) 7/5 lb Permeation data available by calling 877–797–5907 or go to http://www.dupont.com/tyvek/protective-apparel htm.
Applicable Regulations	None
Health Hazards	None
Communications Interface Capability	Not applicable
EOD Compatibility	Compatible with EOD suit

General
Name — *Tychem® QC Shirt*
Item # 22

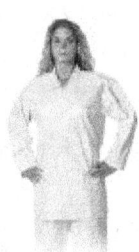

Technology	Selectively impermeable composite consisting of thermoplastic barrier films laminated to high strength thermoplastic nonwoven fabrics
Stock Number	35303
Protection Type	Percutaneous
Equipment Category	Shirt, snap front, and long sleeves
Availability	Commercial
Current User(s)	U.S. Government/military, local government/fire department, emergency response teams, general industry, remediation companies, and chemical manufacturing. Specific organizations currently using item available upon request.
Manufacturer	DuPont Tyvek® Protective Apparel U.S. Highway #1 North McBee, SC 29101 800–845–6962 (Tel) 843–335–8599 (Fax) e-mail: Mary-Ann.Daniel@usa.dupont.com POC: M. A. Daniel 888–577–6960 (Tel)
Manufacturer Type	Domestic manufacturer
Developer	DuPont Protective Apparel
Source	DuPont Tyvek® Protective Apparel
Certification	Not applicable

Operational Parameters

Chemical Warfare (CW) Agents Protected Against	Not tested
Biological Warfare (BW) Agents Protected Against	Not specified
Toxic Industrial (TIMs) Protected Against	Many inorganic acids, bases, and other liquid chemicals such as pesticides. For specific test data, call the DuPont Protective Apparel Fax-on-Demand Service at 800–558–9329 and request document 616, or go to http://www.dupont.com/tyvek/protective-apparel.htm.
Duration of Protection	For specific test data on TIMs, call the DuPont Protective Apparel Fax-on-Demand Service at 800–558–9329 and request document 616, or go to http://www.dupont.com/tyvek/protective-apparel.htm. No test data available for CW agents.
Recommended Use(s)	Crisis management (post decontamination); medical triage; remediation

Physical Parameters

Sizes Available	S through XXXXL. Additional sizes available upon request.
Weight	5 lb/container, 12 units/container
Package Size and Volume	14 7/8 in L x 10 in W x 10 in H
Power Requirements	Not applicable
Material Type	Selectively impermeable composite consisting of thermoplastic barrier films laminated to high strength thermoplastic nonwoven fabrics
Construction Type	Sewn seam—overedge serged seam construction offers protection against many dry particulates and light sprays
Color	Yellow, grey

Logistical Parameters

Ease of Use	Ergonomically designed for maximum mobility and flexibility
Consumables	None
Maintenance Requirements	Visual inspection prior to use
Shelf Life	Store in a cool, dry environment in original packaging. Manufacturer recommends designating "for training use only" after 5 yr of storage.
Transportability	Easily transported
Operational Limitations	Directly relates to the physical condition of user
Environmental Conditions	Can be used in all common outdoor weather conditions and climates. Rain, snow, extreme temperatures and humidity will have no effect on the suit.
Unit Cost	$53/carton
Maintenance Cost	Minimum labor cost for routine suit inspection
Warranty	90 d for workmanship and materials
Don/Doff Information	No assistance required for donning and doffing. Average donning and doffing time is minimal.
Use/Reuse	Discard after use. Decontamination specific to chemical exposure. Disposal per jurisdictional regulations.
Launderability	Not applicable. Not intended for reuse after exposure to toxic chemicals. Dirt and dust can be manually removed with soap and water.
Accessories	None

Special Requirements

Training Requirements	No special training required
Training Available	Yes. DuPont will provide specialized group training upon request.
Manuals Available	Permeation Guide available
Surveillance Testing Requirements	Visual inspection (for holes and tears) prior to use
Support Equipment	Appropriate respiratory, foot, eye/face, hand, and head protection

Testing Information	Physical properties: Basis weight (ASTM D3776–85) 2.1 oz/yd^2 Thickness (ASTM D1777–64) 6.0 mils Mullen burst (ASTM D3786–87) 66 psi Breaking strength—Grab (md/xd) (ASTM D1682–64, sec. 5.3) 25/35 lb Tearing strength—Trapezoid (md/xd) (ASTM D1117–80) 7/5 lb Permeation data available by calling 877–797–5907 or go to http://www.dupont.com/tyvek/protective-apparel.htm.
Applicable Regulations	None
Health Hazards	None
Communications Interface Capability	Not applicable
EOD Compatibility	Compatible with EOD suit

General

Name — *Tychem® QC Pants*

Item # 23

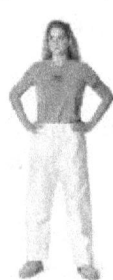

Technology	Selectively impermeable composite consisting of thermoplastic barrier films laminated to high strength thermoplastic nonwoven fabrics
Stock Number	35350
Protection Type	Percutaneous
Equipment Category	Pants, elastic waist
Availability	Commercial
Current User(s)	U.S. Government/military, local government/fire department, emergency response teams, general industry, remediation companies, and chemical manufacturing. Specific organizations currently using item available upon request.
Manufacturer	DuPont Tyvek® Protective Apparel U.S. Highway #1 North McBee, SC 29101 800–845–6962 (Tel) 843–335–8599 (Fax) e-mail: Mary-Ann.Daniel@usa.dupont.com POC: M. A. Daniel 888–577–6960 (Tel)
Manufacturer Type	Domestic manufacturer
Developer	DuPont Protective Apparel
Source	DuPont Tyvek® Protective Apparel
Certification	Not applicable

Operational Parameters

Chemical Warfare (CW) Agents Protected Against	Not tested
Biological Warfare (BW) Agents Protected Against	Not specified
Toxic Industrial (TIMs) Protected Against	Many inorganic acids, bases, and other liquid chemicals such as pesticides. For specific test data, call the DuPont Protective Apparel Fax-on-Demand Service at 800–558–9329 and request document 616, or go to http://www.dupont.com/tyvek/protective-apparel.htm.
Duration of Protection	For specific test data on TIMs, call the DuPont Protective Apparel Fax-on-Demand Service at 800–558–9329 and request document 616, or go to http://www.dupont.com/tyvek/protective-apparel.htm. No test data available for CW agents.
Recommended Use(s)	Crisis management (post decontamination); medical triage; remediation

Physical Parameters

Sizes Available	S through XXXXL. Additional sizes available upon request.
Weight	5 lb/container, 12 units/container
Package Size and Volume	14 7/8 in L x 10 in W x 10 in H
Power Requirements	Not applicable
Material Type	Selectively impermeable composite consisting of thermoplastic barrier films laminated to high strength thermoplastic nonwoven fabrics
Construction Type	Sewn seam—overedge serged seam construction offers protection against many dry particulates and light sprays
Color	Yellow, grey

Logistical Parameters

Ease of Use	Ergonomically designed for maximum mobility and flexibility
Consumables	None
Maintenance Requirements	Visual inspection prior to use
Shelf Life	Store in a cool, dry environment in original packaging. Manufacturer recommends designating "for training use only" after 5 yr of storage.
Transportability	Easily transported
Operational Limitations	Directly relates to the physical condition of user
Environmental Conditions	Can be used in all common outdoor weather conditions and climates. Rain, snow, extreme temperatures and humidity will have no effect on the suit.
Unit Cost	$41/carton
Maintenance Cost	Minimum labor cost for routine suit inspection
Warranty	90 d for workmanship and materials
Don/Doff Information	No assistance required for donning and doffing. Average donning and doffing time is minimal.
Use/Reuse	Discard after use. Decontamination specific to chemical exposure. Disposal per jurisdictional regulations.
Launderability	Not applicable. Not intended for reuse after exposure to toxic chemicals. Dirt and dust can be manually removed with soap and water.
Accessories	None

Special Requirements

Training Requirements	No special training required
Training Available	Yes. DuPont will provide specialized group training upon request.
Manuals Available	Permeation Guide available
Surveillance Testing Requirements	Visual inspection (for holes and tears) prior to use
Support Equipment	Appropriate respiratory, foot, eye/face, hand, and head protection

Testing Information	Physical properties: Basis weight (ASTM D3776–85) 2.1 oz/yd^2 Thickness (ASTM D1777–64) 6.0 mils Mullen burst (ASTM D3786–87) 66 psi Breaking strength—Grab (md/xd) (ASTM D1682–64, sec. 5.3) 25/35 lb Tearing strength—Trapezoid (md/xd) (ASTM D1117–80) 7/5 lb Permeation data available by calling 877–797–5907 or go to http://www.dupont.com/tyvek/protective-apparel htm.
Applicable Regulations	None
Health Hazards	None
Communications Interface Capability	Not applicable
EOD Compatibility	Compatible with EOD suit

General

Name   *Tychem® QC Hood*
Item # 24

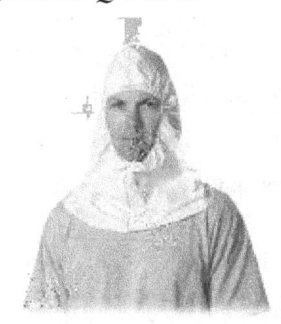

Technology — Selectively impermeable composite consisting of thermoplastic barrier films laminated to high strength thermoplastic nonwoven fabrics

Stock Number — 35386

Protection Type — Percutaneous

Equipment Category — Hood, pull over, shoulder length, and elastic face

Availability — Commercial

Current User(s) — U.S. Government/military, local government/fire department, emergency response teams, general industry, remediation companies, and chemical manufacturing. Specific organizations currently using item available upon request.

Manufacturer — DuPont Tyvek® Protective Apparel
U.S. Highway #1 North
McBee, SC 29101
800–845–6962 (Tel)
843–335–8599 (Fax)
e-mail: Mary-Ann.Daniel@usa.dupont.com
POC: M. A. Daniel
888–577–6960 (Tel)

Manufacturer Type — Domestic manufacturer

Developer — DuPont Protective Apparel

Source — DuPont Tyvek® Protective Apparel

Certification — Not applicable

Operational Parameters

Chemical Warfare (CW) Agents Protected Against — Not tested

Biological Warfare (BW) Agents Protected Against — Not specified

Toxic Industrial (TIMs) Protected Against — Many inorganic acids, bases, and other liquid chemicals such as pesticides. For specific test data, call the DuPont Protective Apparel Fax-on-Demand Service at 800–558–9329 and request document 616, or go to http://www.dupont.com/tyvek/protective-apparel.htm.

Duration of Protection — For specific test data on TIMs, call the DuPont Protective Apparel Fax-on-Demand Sservice at 800–558–9329 and request document 616, or go to http://www.dupont.com/tyvek/protective-apparel.htm. No test data available for CW agents.

Recommended Use(s)	Crisis management (post decontamination); medical triage; and remediation
Physical Parameters	
Sizes Available	S through XXXXL. Additional sizes available upon request.
Weight	3 lb/container, 48 units/container
Package Size and Volume	14 7/8 in L x 10 in W x 10 in H
Power Requirements	Not applicable
Material Type	Selectively impermeable composite consisting of thermoplastic barrier films laminated to high strength thermoplastic nonwoven fabrics
Construction Type	Sewn seam—overedge serged seam construction offers protection against many dry particulates and light sprays
Color	Yellow, grey
Logistical Parameters	
Ease of Use	Ergonomically designed for maximum mobility and flexibility
Consumables	None
Maintenance Requirements	Visual inspection prior to use
Shelf Life	Store in a cool, dry environment in original packaging. Manufacturer recommends designating "for training use only" after 5 yr of storage.
Transportability	Easily transported
Operational Limitations	Directly relates to the physical condition of user
Environmental Conditions	Can be used in all common outdoor weather conditions and climates. Rain, snow, extreme temperatures and humidity will have no effect on the suit.
Unit Cost	$47/carton
Maintenance Cost	Minimum labor cost for routine suit inspection
Warranty	90 d for workmanship and materials
Don/Doff Information	No assistance required for donning and doffing. Average donning and doffing time is minimal.
Use/Reuse	Discard after use. Decontamination specific to chemical exposure. Disposal per jurisdictional regulations.
Launderability	Not applicable. Not intended for reuse after exposure to toxic chemicals. Dirt and dust can be manually removed with soap and water.
Accessories	None
Special Requirements	
Training Requirements	No special training required
Training Available	Yes. DuPont will provide specialized group training upon request.
Manuals Available	Permeation Guide available
Surveillance Testing Requirements	Visual inspection (for holes and tears) prior to use
Support Equipment	Appropriate respiratory, foot, hand, and head protection

Testing Information	Physical properties: Basis weight (ASTM D3776–85) 2.1 oz/yd^2 Thickness (ASTM D1777–64) 6.0 mils Mullen burst (ASTM D3786–87) 66 psi Breaking strength—Grab (md/xd) (ASTM D1682–64, sec. 5.3) 25/35 lb Tearing strength—Trapezoid (md/xd) (ASTM D1117–80) 7/5 lb Permeation data available by calling 877–797–5907 or go to http://www.dupont.com/tyvek/protective-apparel htm.
Applicable Regulations	None
Health Hazards	None
Communications Interface Capability	Not applicable
EOD Compatibility	Compatible with EOD suit

General

Name   *Tychem® QC Hood*
Item # 25

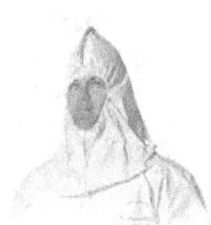

Technology	Selectively impermeable composite consisting of thermoplastic barrier films laminated to high strength thermoplastic nonwoven fabrics
Stock Number	37386
Protection Type	Percutaneous
Equipment Category	Hood, pull over, shoulder length, and elastic face
Availability	Commercial
Current User(s)	U.S. Government/military, local government/fire department, emergency response teams, general industry, remediation companies, and chemical manufacturing. Specific organizations currently using item available upon request.
Manufacturer	DuPont Tyvek® Protective Apparel U.S. Highway #1 North McBee, SC 29101 800–845–6962 (Tel) 843–335–8599 (Fax) e-mail: Mary-Ann.Daniel@usa.dupont.com POC: M. A. Daniel 888–577–6960 (Tel)
Manufacturer Type	Domestic manufacturer
Developer	DuPont Protective Apparel
Source	DuPont Tyvek® Protective Apparel
Certification	Not applicable

Operational Parameters

Chemical Warfare (CW) Agents Protected Against	Not tested
Biological Warfare (BW) Agents Protected Against	Not specified
Toxic Industrial (TIMs) Protected Against	Many inorganic acids, bases, and other liquid chemicals such as pesticides. For specific test data, call the DuPont Protective Apparel Fax-on-Demand Service at 800–558–9329 and request document 616, or go to http://www.dupont.com/tyvek/protective-apparel.htm.
Duration of Protection	For specific test data on TIMs, call the DuPont Protective Apparel Fax-on-Demand Service at 800–558–9329 and request document 616, or go to http://www.dupont.com/tyvek/protective-apparel.htm. No test data available for CW agents.
Recommended Use(s)	Crisis management (post decontamination); medical triage; and remediation

Physical Parameters

Sizes Available	S through XXXXL. Additional sizes available upon request.
Weight	7 lb/container, 48 units/container
Package Size and Volume	14 7/8 in L x 10 in W x 10 in H
Power Requirements	Not applicable
Material Type	Selectively impermeable composite consisting of thermoplastic barrier films laminated to high strength thermoplastic nonwoven fabrics
Construction Type	Bound seam—tightly sewn seam is reinforced with an outer binding to further enhance seam strength and barrier quality
Color	Yellow, grey

Logistical Parameters

Ease of Use	Ergonomically designed for maximum mobility and flexibility
Consumables	None
Maintenance Requirements	Visual inspection prior to use
Shelf Life	Store in a cool, dry environment in original packaging. Manufacturer recommends designating "for training use only" after 5 yr of storage.
Transportability	Easily transported
Operational Limitations	Directly relates to the physical condition of user
Environmental Conditions	Can be used in all common outdoor weather conditions and climates. Rain, snow, extreme temperatures and humidity will have no effect on the suit.
Unit Cost	$54/carton
Maintenance Cost	Minimum labor cost for routine suit inspection
Warranty	90 d for workmanship and materials
Don/Doff Information	No assistance required for donning and doffing. Average donning and doffing time is minimal.
Use/Reuse	Discard after use. Decontamination specific to chemical exposure. Disposal per jurisdictional regulations.
Launderability	Not applicable. Not intended for reuse after exposure to toxic chemicals. Dirt and dust can be manually removed with soap and water.
Accessories	None

Special Requirements

Training Requirements	No special training required
Training Available	Yes. DuPont will provide specialized group training upon request.
Manuals Available	Permeation Guide available
Surveillance Testing Requirements	Visual inspection (for holes and tears) prior to use
Support Equipment	Appropriate respiratory, foot, hand, and head protection

Testing Information	Physical properties: Basis weight (ASTM D3776–85) 2.1 oz/yd^2 Thickness (ASTM D1777–64) 6.0 mils Mullen burst (ASTM D3786–87) 66 psi Breaking strength—Grab (md/xd) (ASTM D1682–64, sec. 5.3) 25/35 lb Tearing strength—Trapezoid (md/xd) (ASTM D1117–80) 7/5 lb Permeation data available by calling 877–797–5907 or go to http://www.dupont.com/tyvek/protective-apparel htm.
Applicable Regulations	None
Health Hazards	None
Communications Interface Capability	Not applicable
EOD Compatibility	Compatible with EOD suit

General

Name *Tychem® SL Hood*

Item # 26

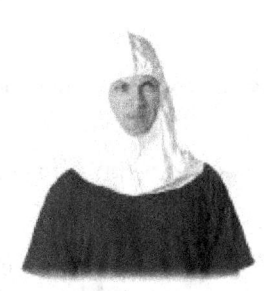

Technology	Selectively impermeable composite consisting of thermoplastic barrier films laminated to high strength thermoplastic nonwoven fabrics
Stock Number	42386
Protection Type	Percutaneous
Equipment Category	Hood, hood, elastic face, pull over, and shoulder length
Availability	Commercial
Current User(s)	U.S. Government/military, local government/fire department, emergency response teams, general industry, remediation companies, and chemical manufacturing. Specific organizations currently using item available upon request.
Manufacturer	DuPont Tyvek® Protective Apparel U.S. Highway #1 North McBee, SC 29101 800–845–6962 (Tel) 843–335–8599 (Fax) e-mail: Mary-Ann.Daniel@usa.dupont.com POC: M. A. Daniel 888–577–6960 (Tel)
Manufacturer Type	Domestic manufacturer
Developer	DuPont Protective Apparel
Source	DuPont Tyvek® Protective Apparel
Certification	Not applicable

Operational Parameters

Chemical Warfare (CW) Agents Protected Against	Nerve agents (GB and VX); blister agents (HD and L). For specific test results, call the DuPont Protective Apparel Fax-on-Demand Service at 800–558–9329 and request Document 595.
Biological Warfare (BW) Agents Protected Against	Not specified
Toxic Industrial (TIMs) Protected Against	A broad range of liquid chemicals. For specific test data, call the DuPont Protective Apparel Fax-on-Demand Service at 800–558–9329 and request document 621, or go to http://www.dupont.com/tyvek/protective-apparel.htm.
Duration of Protection	Fabric test data: Average breakthrough time VX: Greater than 12 h at 10 g/m^2 GB, and L: Greater than 6 h at 10 g/m^2 D: Greater than 3 h at 10 g/m^2

For specific test data on TIMs, call the DuPont Protective Apparel Fax-on-Demand Service at 800–558–9329.

Recommended Use(s)	Crisis management; remediation; and decontamination
Physical Parameters	
Sizes Available	S through XXXXL. Additional sizes available upon request.
Weight	5 lb/container, 48 unit/container
Package Size and Volume	14 7/8 in L x 10 in W x 10 in H
Power Requirements	Not applicable
Material Type	Selectively impermeable composite consisting of thermoplastic barrier films laminated to high strength thermoplastic nonwoven fabrics
Construction Type	Bound seam—tightly sew seam is reinforced with an outer binding to further enhance seam strength and barrier quality
Color	White
Logistical Parameters	
Ease of Use	Ergonomically designed for maximum mobility and flexibility
Consumables	None
Maintenance Requirements	Visual inspection prior to use
Shelf Life	Store in a cool, dry environment in original packaging. Manufacturer recommends designating "for training use only" after 5 yr of storage.
Transportability	Easily transported
Operational Limitations	Directly relates to the physical condition of user
Environmental Conditions	Can be used in all common outdoor weather conditions and climates. Rain, snow, extreme temperatures and humidity will have no effect on the suit.
Unit Cost	$89/carton
Maintenance Cost	Minimum labor cost for routine suit inspection
Warranty	90 d for workmanship and materials
Don/Doff Information	No assistance required for donning and doffing. Average donning and doffing time is minimal.
Use/Reuse	Discard after use. Decontamination specific to chemical exposure. Disposal per jurisdictional regulations.
Launderability	Not applicable. Not intended for reuse after exposure to toxic chemicals. Dirt and dust can be manually removed with soap and water.
Accessories	None
Special Requirements	
Training Requirements	No special training required
Training Available	Yes. DuPont will provide specialized group training upon request.
Manuals Available	Permeation Guide available
Surveillance Testing Requirements	Visual inspection (for holes and tears) prior to use

Support Equipment	Appropriate respiratory, foot, hand, and head protection
Testing Information	Physical properties: Basis weight (ASTM D3776–85) 3.1 oz/yd^2 Thickness (ASTM D1777–64) 10.3 mils Mullen burst (ASTM D3786–87) 78 psi Breaking strength—Grab (md/xd) (ASTM D1682–64, sec. 5.3) 42/45 lb Tearing strength—Trapezoid (md/xd) (ASTM D1117–80) 11/9 lb Permeation data available by calling 877–797–5907 or go to http://www.dupont.com/tyvek/protective-apparel htm.
Applicable Regulations	None
Health Hazards	None
Communications Interface Capability	Not applicable
EOD Compatibility	Compatible with EOD suit

General
Name — *Tychem® BR Hood/Vest*
Item # 27

Technology — Selectively impermeable composite consisting of thermoplastic barrier films laminated to high strength thermoplastic nonwoven fabrics

Stock Number — 95389

Protection Type — Percutaneous

Equipment Category — Hood/vest, pullover, PVC face shield, and velcro waist belt

Availability — Commercial

Current User(s) — U.S. Government/military, local government/fire department, emergency response teams, general industry, remediation companies, and chemical manufacturing. Specific organizations currently using item available upon request.

Manufacturer — DuPont Tyvek® Protective Apparel
U.S. Highway #1 North
McBee, SC 29101
800–845–6962 (Tel)
843–335–8599 (Fax)
e-mail: Mary-Ann.Daniel@usa.dupont.com
POC: M. A. Daniel
888–577–6960 (Tel)

Manufacturer Type — Domestic manufacturer

Developer — DuPont Protective Apparel

Source — DuPont Tyvek® Protective Apparel

Certification — Not applicable

Operational Parameters
Chemical Warfare (CW) Agents Protected Against — Nerve agents (GA, GB, GD, and VX); blister agents (HD and L). For specific test results, call the DuPont Protective Apparel Fax-on-Demand Service at 800–558–9329 and request Document 595.

Biological Warfare (BW) Agents Protected Against — Not specified

Toxic Industrial (TIMs) Protected Against — A broad range of TIMs. For specific test data, call the DuPont Protective Apparel Fax-on-Demand Service at 800–558–9329 and request document 648, or go to http://www.dupont.com/tyvek/protective-apparel.htm.

Duration of Protection	Fabric test data: Average breakthrough time GA, GB, GD, HD, L, and VX: Greater than 12 h at 10 g/m^2 GB, HD, and VX: Greater than 12 h at 100 g/m^2 (total coverage) L: Greater than 2 h at 100 g/m2 (total coverage) For specific test data on TIMs, call the DuPont Protective Apparel Fax-on-Demand Service at 800–558–9329 and request document 636, or go to http://www.dupont.com/tyvek/protective-apparel.htm.
Recommended Use(s)	Emergency response; crisis management; remediation, secondary decontamination in hospital or emergency area, and warm zone decontamination

Physical Parameters

Sizes Available	S through XXXXL. Additional sizes available upon request.
Weight	3 lb/container, 2 units/container
Package Size and Volume	16 in L x 10 1/4 in W x 14 1/8 in H
Power Requirements	Not applicable
Material Type	Selectively impermeable composite consisting of thermoplastic barrier films laminated to high strength thermoplastic nonwoven fabrics
Construction Type	Thermo Bond Seam—sewn and taped. This exceptionally strong and chemical resistant seam construction provides a reliable barrier against heavy liquid splashes and rigorous seam stress
Color	Yellow or olive drab

Logistical Parameters

Ease of Use	Ergonomically designed for maximum mobility and flexibility
Consumables	None
Maintenance Requirements	Visual inspection prior to use
Shelf Life	Store in a cool, dry environment in original packaging. Manufacturer recommends designating "for training use only" after 5 yr of storage.
Transportability	Easily transported
Operational Limitations	Directly relates to the physical condition of user
Environmental Conditions	Can be used in all common outdoor weather conditions and climates. Rain, snow, extreme temperatures and humidity will have no effect on the suit.
Unit Cost	$75/carton
Maintenance Cost	Minimum labor cost for routine suit inspection
Warranty	90 d for workmanship and materials
Don/Doff Information	No assistance required for donning and doffing. Average donning and doffing time is minimal.
Use/Reuse	Discard after use. Decontamination specific to chemical exposure. Disposal per jurisdictional regulations.
Launderability	Not applicable. Not intended for reuse after exposure to toxic chemicals. Dirt and dust can be manually removed with soap and water.

Accessories None

Special Requirements

Training Requirements No special training required

Training Available Yes. DuPont will provide specialized group training upon request.

Manuals Available Permeation Guide available

Surveillance Testing Requirements Visual inspection (for holes and tears) prior to use

Support Equipment Appropriate respiratory, foot, hand, and head protection

Testing Information Physical properties:
Basis weight (ASTM D3776–85) 6.6 oz/yd^2
Thickness (ASTM D1777–64) 16 mils
Ball burst (ASTM D3787–89) 90 psi
Breaking strength—Grab (md/xd) (ASTM D5034) 90/84 lb
Tearing strength—Trapezoid (md/xd) (ASTM D5597) 19/19 lb
Permeation data available by calling 877–797–5907 or go to http://www.dupont.com/tyvek/protective-apparel.htm.

Applicable Regulations None

Health Hazards None

Communications Interface Capability Not applicable

EOD Compatibility Compatible with EOD suit

General

Name — *Tychem® TK Hood/Vest*
Item # 28

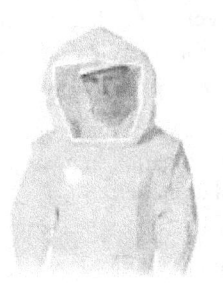

Technology — Selectively impermeable composite consisting of thermoplastic barrier films laminated to high strength thermoplastic nonwoven fabrics

Stock Number — TK389

Protection Type — Percutaneous

Equipment Category — Hood/vest, pullover, PVC face shield, and velcro waist belt

Availability — Commercial

Current User(s) — U.S. Government/military, local government/fire department, emergency response teams, general industry, remediation companies, and chemical manufacturing. Specific organizations currently using item available upon request.

Manufacturer — DuPont Tyvek® Protective Apparel
U.S. Highway #1 North
McBee, SC 29101
800–845–6962 (Tel)
843–335–8599 (Fax)
e-mail: Mary-Ann.Daniel@usa.dupont.com
POC: M. A. Daniel
888–577–6960 (Tel)

Manufacturer Type — Domestic manufacturer

Developer — DuPont Protective Apparel

Source — DuPont Tyvek® Protective Apparel

Certification — Not applicable

Operational Parameters

Chemical Warfare (CW) Agents Protected Against — Nerve agents (GA, GB, GD, and VX); blister agents (HD and L). For specific test results, call the DuPont Protective Apparel Fax-on-Demand Service at 800–558–9329 and request Document 595.

Biological Warfare (BW) Agents Protected Against — Not specified

Toxic Industrial (TIMs) Protected Against — Excellent protection against a wide variety of TIMs. For specific test data, call the DuPont Protective Apparel Fax-on-Demand service at 800–558–9329 and request document 651, or go to http://www.dupont.com/tyvek/protective-apparel.htm.

Duration of Protection	Fabric test data: Average breakthrough time GB, HD, VX, and L: Greater than 12 h at 100 g/m^2 (total coverage) GA, GB, GD, HD, L, and VX: Greater than 12 h at 10 g/m^2 For specific test data on TIMs, call the DuPont Protective Apparel Fax-on-Demand Service at 800–558–9329 and request document 651, or go to http://www.dupont.com/tyvek/protective-apparel.htm.
Recommended Use(s)	Emergency response; crisis management; remediation, secondary decontamination in hospital or emergency area, and warm zone decontamination

Physical Parameters

Sizes Available	S through XXXXL. Additional sizes available upon request.
Weight	3 lb/container, 2 units/container
Package Size and Volume	16 in L x 10 1/4 in W x 14 1/8 in H
Power Requirements	Not applicable
Material Type	Selectively impermeable composite consisting of thermoplastic barrier films laminated to high strength thermoplastic nonwoven fabrics
Construction Type	Thermo bond seam—sewn and taped. This exceptionally strong and chemical resistant seam construction provides a reliable barrier against heavy liquid splashes and rigorous seam stress.
Color	High-visibility lime yellow

Logistical Parameters

Ease of Use	Ergonomically designed for maximum mobility and flexibility
Consumables	None
Maintenance Requirements	Visual inspection prior to use
Shelf Life	Store in a cool, dry environment in original packaging. Manufacturer recommends designating "for training use only" after 5 yr of storage.
Transportability	Easily transported
Operational Limitations	Directly relates to the physical condition of user
Environmental Conditions	Can be used in all common outdoor weather conditions and climates. Rain, snow, extreme temperatures and humidity will have no effect on the suit.
Unit Cost	$83/carton
Maintenance Cost	Minimum labor cost for routine suit inspection
Warranty	90 d for workmanship and materials
Don/Doff Information	No assistance required for donning and doffing. Average donning and doffing time is minimal.
Use/Reuse	Discard after use. Decontamination specific to chemical exposure. Disposal per jurisdictional regulations.
Launderability	Not applicable. Not intended for reuse after exposure to toxic chemicals. Dirt and dust can be manually removed with soap and water.

Accessories None

Special Requirements
Training Requirements No special training required

Training Available Yes. DuPont will provide specialized group training upon request.

Manuals Available Permeation Guide available

Surveillance Testing Requirements Visual inspection (for holes and tears) prior to use

Support Equipment Appropriate respiratory, foot, hand, and head protection

Testing Information Physical properties:
Basis weight (ASTM D3776) 10.6 oz/yd^2
Thickness (ASTM D1777) 26 mils
Ball burst (ASTM D3787) 187 psi
Breaking strength—Grab (md/xd) (ASTM D15034) 188/180 lb
Tearing strength—Trapezoid (md/xd) (ASTM D5733) 53/52 lb
Permeation data available by calling 877–797–5907 or go to http://www.dupont.com/tyvek/protective-apparel.htm.

Applicable Regulations None

Health Hazards None

Communications Interface Capability Not applicable

EOD Compatibility Compatible with EOD suit

General

Name — *Integrated Chemical Biological Protective Glove*
Item # 29

Picture Not Available

Technology — Permeable oil/water repellant outer fabric with leather palm and integrated CB interior filter material with bonded face. Standard model not fire resistant (FR); FR model available (different outer material).

Stock Number — ICBPG-S: Standard. Glove; ICBPG-F: FR Glove

Protection Type — Skin protection from Military Chemical/Biological warfare agents

Equipment Category — Five finger protective glove with gauntlet, offering high dexterity and comfort

Availability — Standard Med—60 d after order
FR Model—90 d to 120 d after order

Current User(s) — Field tested for NATO Military use

Manufacturer — Wells Lamont

Manufacturer Type — Private, Foreign/USA

Developer — Gants Rigaudy

Source — Sales: INDEF Services Intl
14847 Lee Highway
Amissville, VA 20106–0089
540–937–7327 (Tel)
540–937–7328 (Fax)
e-mail: indefsteve@msn.com

Certification — Meets NATO Military Standard

Operational Parameters

Chemical Warfare (CW) Agents Protected Against — All Military CW agents

Biological Warfare (BW) Agents Protected Against — All Military BW agents

Toxic Industrial (TIMs) Protected Against — Not applicable

Duration of Protection — Minimum 8 h against NATO standard challenge

Recommended Use(s) — Tactical operations, CBW response teams: Used with CB Protective Ensemble by ground personnel, air crews, and vehicle operators. Particularly designed where high dexterity and comfort are required.

Physical Parameters

Sizes Available — S, M, L, and XL

Weight — 14 oz

Package Size and Volume — 16 in x 6 in x 1.5 in—0.1 cuff

Power Requirements — None

Material Type — Permeable oil/water repellant outer fabric with leather palm and integrated CB interior filter material with bonded face. Standard model not FR; FR model available (different outer material).

Construction Type	Sewn
Color	Forest green or tan
Logistical Parameters	
Ease of Use	Simple pull on—no training required. Gloves provide maximum comfort (even in hot/humid) and optimum dexterity (ease of picking up objects and handling).
Consumables	None
Maintenance Requirements	None
Shelf Life	Estimated 6 yr to 8 yr
Transportability	Not applicable
Operational Limitations	Not for use with industrial HazMat
Environmental Conditions	-30 °F to +140 °F. Maintains protection if wet.
Unit Cost	$70/pair
Maintenance Cost	None
Warranty	Replacement if manufacturing flaw found upon initial use within 12 mo of purchase.
Don/Doff Information	Glove is worn over skin with gauntlet over arm of ensemble. Can be don without assistance.
Use/Reuse	Use minimum 14 d in normal wear
Launderability	Hand wash only up to 3 times (inspect for tears/wear after each)
Accessories	None
Special Requirements	
Training Requirements	None
Training Available	None required
Manuals Available	None required
Surveillance Testing Requirements	Recommend periodic test of sample from each lot after 24 mo to 36 mo
Support Equipment	None
Testing Information	Meets NATO Standard Test Requirement for CB ensemble
Applicable Regulations	Not applicable
Health Hazards	None
Communications Interface Capability	Not applicable
EOD Compatibility	Yes

General

Name — *NBC Gloves*

Item # 30

Picture Not Available

Technology — Rolamit-NBC Barrierfilm—A 7–layer polyolefin film laminated in staggered angles with 3 layers on either side with a middle barrier of EVOH; impermeable; self-extinguishing

Stock Number — Sweden Civil Defense nsn 12881

Protection Type — Not specified

Equipment Category — Gloves

Availability — In production since 1987

Current User(s) — Swedish Civil Defense

Manufacturer — Goetzloff GmbH
Schirmerstrasse 28, A–4060
Leonding-Linz, Austria
POC: Mr. Lewis B. Sykes (U.S. Liaison)
703–504–0260 (Tel)
e-mail: LBS1328@aol.com

Manufacturer Type — Foreign

Developer — Goetzloff GmbH

Source — Goetzloff GmbH

Certification — Ministry of Defense, Austria

Operational Parameters

Chemical Warfare (CW) Agents Protected Against — Classical nerve and blister agents; test documents can be supplied on request

Biological Warfare (BW) Agents Protected Against — Classical BW agents; test documents can be supplied on request

Toxic Industrial (TIMs) Protected Against — TIMs tested according ASTM F 1001

Duration of Protection — Depends on the situation; e.g., in excess of 24 h against Mustard in worst-case scenarios

Recommended Use(s) — Tactical and crisis management

Physical Parameters

Sizes Available — S, M, L, and XL

Weight — 1 oz per pair

Package Size and Volume — 16.2 in

Power Requirements — None

Material Type — Rolamit-NBC barrierfilm—A 7–layer polyolefin film laminated in staggered angles with 3 layers on either side with a middle barrier of EVOH; impermeable; self-extinguishing

Construction Type — Yes; heat sealed

Color — Standard color is military green, other colors on request

Logistical Parameters

Ease of Use	User has complete freedom of movement; glove has three fingers
Consumables	None
Maintenance Requirements	None
Shelf Life	Indefinite when stored in original wrapper
Transportability	Not applicable
Operational Limitations	Not specified
Environmental Conditions	Designed to be worn under common environmental conditions found in the field
Unit Cost	$1.50 per pair
Maintenance Cost	None
Warranty	20 yr in unconditioned storage
Don/Doff Information	No assistance required for donning or doffing
Use/Reuse	Reusable
Launderability	Can be laundered multiple times with standard detergents and maintain their effectiveness; standard decon procedures can be used
Accessories	None

Special Requirements

Training Requirements	None
Training Available	None required
Manuals Available	None required
Surveillance Testing Requirements	Visual inspection before and after each use
Support Equipment	None
Testing Information	Test data can be obtained on request
Applicable Regulations	Our products are tested by TNO, which certifies NATO standard for our products
Health Hazards	None; incineration results in no toxic residues
Communications Interface Capability	Not specified
EOD Compatibility	Not specified

General

Name — *Eurolite NBC-Casualty Bag*

Item # 31

Picture Not Available

Technology — Rolamit-NBC Barrierfilm—A 7–layer polyolefin film laminated in staggered angles with 3 layers on either side with a middle barrier of EVOH; impermeable; self-extinguishing

Stock Number — ZABCCASBAG

Protection Type — Not specified

Equipment Category — Casualty bag

Availability — In production since 1995

Current User(s) — Austrian Army

Manufacturer — Goetzloff GmbH
Schirmerstrasse 28, A–4060
Leonding-Linz, Austria
POC: Mr. Lewis B. Sykes (U.S. Liaison)
703–504–0260 (Tel)
e-mail: LBS1328@aol.com

Manufacturer Type — Foreign

Developer — Goetzloff GmbH

Source — Goetzloff GmbH

Certification — Ministry of Defense, Austria

Operational Parameters

Chemical Warfare (CW) Agents Protected Against — Classical nerve and blister agents; test documents can be supplied on request

Biological Warfare (BW) Agents Protected Against — Classical BW agents; test documents can be supplied on request

Toxic Industrial (TIMs) Protected Against — TIMs tested according ASTM F 1001

Duration of Protection — Depends on the situation; e.g., in excess of 24 h against Mustard in worst-case scenarios

Recommended Use(s) — Tactical and crisis management

Physical Parameters

Sizes Available — S, M, L, and XL

Weight — 23 oz

Package Size and Volume — 30 in x 25 in x 4 in

Power Requirements — None

Material Type — Rolamit-NBC barrierfilm—A 7–layer polyolefin film laminated in staggered angles with 3 layers on either side with a middle barrier of EVOH; impermeable; self-extinguishing

Construction Type — Yes; heat sealed

Color — Standard color is military green, other colors on request

Logistical Parameters

Ease of Use	User has complete freedom of movement; glove has three fingers
Consumables	None
Maintenance Requirements	None
Shelf Life	Indefinite when stored in original wrapper
Transportability	Not applicable
Operational Limitations	Not specified
Environmental Conditions	Designed to be worn under common environmental conditions found in the field
Unit Cost	$70
Maintenance Cost	None
Warranty	20 yr in unconditioned storage
Don/Doff Information	No assistance required for donning or doffing
Use/Reuse	Reusable
Launderability	Can be laundered multiple times with standard detergents and maintain their effectiveness; standard decon procedures can be used
Accessories	Blowing unit

Special Requirements

Training Requirements	None
Training Available	None required
Manuals Available	None required
Surveillance Testing Requirements	Visual inspection before and after each use
Support Equipment	None
Testing Information	Test data can be obtained on request
Applicable Regulations	Our products are tested by TNO, which certifies NATO standard for our products
Health Hazards	None; incineration results in no toxic residues
Communications Interface Capability	Not specified
EOD Compatibility	Not specified

General
Name *Eurolite NBC-Cover Poncho*
Item # 32

Picture Not Available

Technology Rolamit-NBC Barrierfilm—A 7–layer polyolefin film laminated in staggered angles with 3 layers on either side with a middle barrier of EVOH; impermeable; self-extinguishing

Stock Number ZABCCCPBSF
Protection Type Not specified
Equipment Category Poncho
Availability In production since 1987
Current User(s) Austrian Army, Swedish Civil Defense
Manufacturer Goetzloff GmbH
Schirmerstrasse 28, A–4060
Leonding-Linz, Austria
POC: Mr. Lewis B. Sykes (U.S. Liaison)
703–504–0260 (Tel)
e-mail: LBS1328@aol.com

Manufacturer Type Foreign
Developer Goetzloff GmbH
Source Goetzloff GmbH
Certification Ministry of Defense, Austria

Operational Parameters
Chemical Warfare (CW) Agents Protected Against Classical nerve and blister agents; test documents can be supplied on request
Biological Warfare (BW) Agents Protected Against Classical BW agents; test documents can be supplied on request
Toxic Industrial (TIMs) Protected Against TIMs tested according ASTM F 1001
Duration of Protection Depends on the situation; e.g., in excess of 24 h against Mustard in worst-case scenarios
Recommended Use(s) Tactical and crisis management

Physical Parameters
Sizes Available S, M, L, and XL
Weight 8.8 oz
Package Size and Volume 13 in x 11in x 4 in
Power Requirements None
Material Type Rolamit-NBC barrierfilm—A 7–layer polyolefin film laminated in staggered angles with 3 layers on either side with a middle barrier of EVOH; impermeable; self-extinguishing
Construction Type Yes; heat sealed
Color Standard color is military green, other colors on request

Logistical Parameters

Ease of Use	User has complete freedom of movement; glove has three fingers
Consumables	None
Maintenance Requirements	None
Shelf Life	Indefinite when stored in original wrapper
Transportability	Not applicable
Operational Limitations	Not specified
Environmental Conditions	Designed to be worn under common environmental conditions found in the field
Unit Cost	$6
Maintenance Cost	None
Warranty	20 yr in unconditioned storage
Don/Doff Information	No assistance required for donning or doffing
Use/Reuse	Reusable
Launderability	Can be laundered multiple times with standard detergents and maintain their effectiveness; standard decon procedures can be used
Accessories	None

Special Requirements

Training Requirements	None
Training Available	None required
Manuals Available	None required
Surveillance Testing Requirements	Visual inspection before and after each use
Support Equipment	None
Testing Information	Test data can be obtained on request
Applicable Regulations	Our products are tested by TNO, which certifies NATO standard for our products
Health Hazards	None; incineration results in no toxic residues
Communications Interface Capability	Not specified
EOD Compatibility	Not specified

General

Name *Chemical Protective Butyl Rubber Gloves*

Item # 33

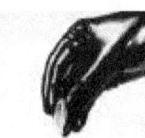

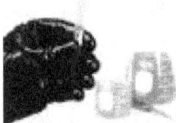

Technology	Guardian gloves are "solution-dipped," providing unparalleled protection for their users. Tight molecular structures are the key to chemical impermeability. Our state-of-the-art microprocessors provide accurate controls every step of the way, from mixing our proprietary compounds, to dipping, curing and drying, in order to attain the necessary strength.
Stock Number	(CP–14F, CP–14FR, and CP–7F)
Protection Type	Percutaneous
Equipment Category	Gloves, CP–14, Surgical Fit Gloves
Availability	Commercial
Current User(s)	U.S. Government (DLA)
Manufacturer	Guardian Manufacturing Co. 302 Conwell Ave. Willard, OH 44890–9529 POC: Gene Lamoreaux 419–933–2711 (Tel) 419–935–8961 (Fax) 800–243–7379 (Tel) e-mail: susanl@willard-oh.com http://www.guardian-mfg.com
Manufacturer Type	Domestic
Developer	Guardian
Source	Internet: http://www.guardian-mfg.com/guardianmfg.html
Certification	ISO–9001 Registered, Defense Supply Center, Philadelphia, PA

Operational Parameters

Chemical Warfare (CW) Agents Protected Against	All
Biological Warfare (BW) Agents Protected Against	All
Toxic Industrial (TIMs) Protected Against	Same chemical protection properties as standard line of Butyl Gloves. Acids, alkalis, MEK, MIBK, acetone, others
Duration of Protection	Mustard resistance 240 min. GB resistance 450 min.
Recommended Use(s)	Industrial, laboratory, first response, and chemical production

Physical Parameters

Sizes Available	XS to XL (5 sizes)
Weight	3.5 lb per dozen pairs
Package Size and Volume	16 in x 6.5 in x 4 in
Power Requirements	Not applicable
Material Type	Butyl—Impermeable
Construction Type	Seamless—Manufactured on a surgical form in 7 mil and 14 mil thickness. Finish is either smooth or rough. The medium weight style, CP–14FR, is available with a pumice overdip for greater grip capability. The additional pumice dip provides a glove which meets or exceeds the permeation capabilities of the smooth style.
Color	Black

Logistical Parameters

Ease of Use	Designed for comfort, security, and dexterity
Consumables	Not applicable
Maintenance Requirements	Not applicable
Shelf Life	5 yr
Transportability	Not applicable
Operational Limitations	Not applicable
Environmental Conditions	Not applicable
Unit Cost	$9.39 per pair
Maintenance Cost	Not applicable
Warranty	5 yr
Don/Doff Information	Not applicable
Use/Reuse	Gloves can be decontaminated with Super Tropical Bleach (STB)
Launderability	Unknown
Accessories	Not applicable

Special Requirements

Training Requirements	Minimal
Training Available	Not applicable
Manuals Available	Not applicable
Surveillance Testing Requirements	Not applicable
Support Equipment	Not applicable
Testing Information	Meets requirements of MIL–G–43976
Applicable Regulations	MIL–G–43976
Health Hazards	None
Communications Interface Capability	Meets requirements of MIL–G–43976
EOD Compatibility	Compatible with current suits

General

Name: *Chemical Protective Butyl Rubber Gloves*

Item # 34

Technology: Guardian gloves are "solution-dipped," providing unparalleled protection for their users. Tight molecular structures are the key to chemical impermeability. Our state-of-the-art microprocessors provide accurate controls every step of the way, from mixing our proprietary compounds, to dipping, curing and drying, in order to attain the necessary strength.

Stock Number: CP-25

Protection Type: Percutaneous

Equipment Category: Gloves

Availability: Commercial

Current User(s): U.S. Government (DLA)

Manufacturer: Guardian Manufacturing Co.
302 Conwell Ave.
Willard, OH 44890-9529
POC: Gene Lamoreaux
419-933-2711 (Tel)
419-935-8961 (Fax)
800-243-7379 (Tel)
e-mail: susanl@willard-oh.com
http://www.guardian-mfg.com

Manufacturer Type: Domestic

Developer: Guardian

Source: Internet: http://www.guardian-mfg.com/guardianmfg.html

Certification: ISO-9001 Registered
ASTM F739-85 by TRI/Environmental, Inc.
Manufactured according to Mil-G-43976, Mil-G-12223, and ZZ-G-381, Defense Supply Center, Philadelphia, PA

Operational Parameters

Chemical Warfare (CW) Agents Protected Against: All

Biological Warfare (BW) Agents Protected Against: All

Toxic Industrial (TIMs) Protected Against: Same chemical protection properties as standard line of Butyl Gloves. Acids, alkalis, MEK, MIBK, acetone, and others.

Duration of Protection: Mustard resistance 360 min. GB resistance 450 min.

Recommended Use(s): Industrial, laboratory, first response, and chemical production

Physical Parameters

Sizes Available	XS to SL (5 sizes)
Weight	5 lb per dozen pairs
Package Size and Volume	16 in x 6.5 in x 6 in
Power Requirements	Not applicable
Material Type	Butyl—impermeable. Available in four thicknesses.
Construction Type	Seamless—The rough-grip finish, gives increased dexterity and improved grip. It is now available on Guardian lightweight butyl. Guardian also offers the rough-grip finish on its medium and heavyweight Butyl gloves.
Color	Black

Logistical Parameters

Ease of Use	Not specified
Consumables	Not applicable
Maintenance Requirements	Not applicable
Shelf Life	5 yr
Transportability	Not applicable
Operational Limitations	Not applicable
Environmental Conditions	Not applicable
Unit Cost	$16.71 per pair
Maintenance Cost	Not applicable
Warranty	5 yr
Don/Doff Information	Not applicable
Use/Reuse	Gloves can be decontaminated with STB
Launderability	Unknown
Accessories	Not applicable

Special Requirements

Training Requirements	Minimal
Training Available	Not applicable
Manuals Available	Not applicable
Surveillance Testing Requirements	Not applicable
Support Equipment	Not applicable
Testing Information	Meets requirements of MIL-G-43976
Applicable Regulations	MIL-G-43976
Health Hazards	None
Communications Interface Capability	Not applicable
EOD Compatibility	Compatible with current suits

General

Name — *Neoprene Gloves*

Item # 35

Technology — Guardian gloves are "solution-dipped," providing unparalleled protection for their users. Tight molecular structures are the key to chemical impermeability. Our state-of-the-art microprocessors provide accurate controls every step of the way, from mixing our proprietary compounds, to dipping, curing and drying, in order to attain the necessary strength.

Stock Number — Not specified

Protection Type — Percutaneous

Equipment Category — Gloves (vapor protection when properly worn as part of the glove system with the complete vapor protective garment ensemble)

Availability — Commercial

Current User(s) — Not specified

Manufacturer — Guardian Manufacturing Co.
302 Conwell Ave.
Willard, OH 44890–9529
POC: Gene Lamoreaux
419–933–2711 (Tel)
419–935–8961 (Fax)
800–243–7379 (Tel)
e-mail: susanl@willard-oh.com
http://www.guardian-mfg.com

Manufacturer Type — Domestic

Developer — Guardian

Source — Internet: http://www.guardian-mfg.com/guardianmfg.html

Certification — ISO–9001 Registered.
Manufactured according to ZZ–G–381.
NFPA 1992—Splash protection.
NFPA 1991—Vapor protection garment specification.

Operational Parameters

Chemical Warfare (CW) Agents Protected Against — Yes

Biological Warfare (BW) Agents Protected Against — Not specified

Toxic Industrial (TIMs) Protected Against — Yes

Duration of Protection — Not specified

E–86
ID# 35

Recommended Use(s)	Provide chemical protection and resist deterioration from contact with petroleum products
Physical Parameters	
Sizes Available	9, 10, 11, and 12
Weight	Not specified
Package Size and Volume	Not specified
Power Requirements	None
Material Type	Neoprene. Guardian meets the needs of tomorrow, today with a sophisticated Research and Development facility complete with research laboratory and a mini-factory where new compounds and processes are tested daily. Guardian gloves will exceed your expectations in comfort, utility, and design.
Construction Type	Smooth finish
Color	Black
Logistical Parameters	
Ease of Use	Not specified
Consumables	Not applicable
Maintenance Requirements	None
Shelf Life	Not specified
Transportability	Not applicable
Operational Limitations	Not applicable
Environmental Conditions	Not specified
Unit Cost	Not specified
Maintenance Cost	None
Warranty	Not specified
Don/Doff Information	No assistance necessary
Use/Reuse	Reusable
Launderability	Not specified
Accessories	None
Special Requirements	
Training Requirements	None
Training Available	Not applicable
Manuals Available	Not applicable
Surveillance Testing Requirements	Not applicable
Support Equipment	Not applicable
Testing Information	Not specified
Applicable Regulations	Not specified
Health Hazards	None
Communications Interface Capability	Meets requirements of MIL-G-43976
EOD Compatibility	Not specified

General

Name	*NBC Casualty Bag*
Item # 36	
	Picture Not Available
Technology	Charcoal impregnated inner. Liquid chemical resistant outer fabric. Vinyl coated lower section.
Stock Number	ID–111–100
Protection Type	Percutaneous
Equipment Category	Casualty bag
Availability	In production
Current User(s)	Earlier version used by Canadian Department of National Defense
Manufacturer	Irvin Aerospace Canada Ltd. P.O. Box 280 479 Central Avenue Fort Erie, Ontario L2A 5M9 POC: Doug Eaton 905–871–6510 (Tel) 905–871–6534 (Fax)
Manufacturer Type	Foreign
Developer	Irvin Aerospace Canada Ltd., with support of Canadian Department of National Defense
Source	Irvin Aerospace Canada Ltd., with support of Canadian Department of National Defense
Certification	Canadian Department of National Defense

Operational Parameters

Chemical Warfare (CW) Agents Protected Against	All known military chemical agents
Biological Warfare (BW) Agents Protected Against	None
Toxic Industrial (TIMs) Protected Against	Under study
Duration of Protection	24 h (in most cases)
Recommended Use(s)	Not specified

Physical Parameters

Sizes Available	Not applicable
Weight	26 lb
Package Size and Volume	24 in x 24 in x 8 in
Power Requirements	12 V dc battery pack (provided as option)
Material Type	Charcoal impregnated inner. Liquid chemical resistant outer fabric. Vinyl coated lower section.
Construction Type	Sewn and sealed as required
Color	Per customer requirements

Logistical Parameters

Ease of Use	Fast closing and opening
Consumables	Canisters
Maintenance Requirements	Routine preventative maintenance
Shelf Life	10 yr minimum
Transportability	Fully transportable
Operational Limitations	Full military qualification
Environmental Conditions	All common military environmental conditions
Unit Cost	Approximately $1.85K without blower assembly, depending upon configuration. Volume dependant.
Maintenance Cost	Not applicable
Warranty	1 yr
Don/Doff Information	Casualty requires assistance to enter and exit
Use/Reuse	Reusable
Launderability	Laundering: clean in soapy water. Decontamination: operator dependent
Accessories	Blower, canisters, and battery pack

Special Requirements

Training Requirements	1 h
Training Available	Yes. Operator and trainer courses available.
Manuals Available	User, maintenance, and repair
Surveillance Testing Requirements	Visual inspection
Support Equipment	Battery pack and batteries for blower
Testing Information	Available from Irvin Aerospace Canada Ltd.
Applicable Regulations	Not applicable
Health Hazards	Not applicable
Communications Interface Capability	Not applicable
EOD Compatibility	Not specified

General

Name *Kappler CPF 4 Bib Overall*

Item # 37

Picture Not Available

Technology Multi-layer barrier film composite laminated to a high strength 2.3 oz polypropylene substrate

Stock Number 4T459

Protection Type Percutaneous

Equipment Category Overalls—adjustable webbing straps and snap lock closures

Availability In stock

Current User(s) REC's Customers: EPA; Department of State Consequence Management & Diplomatic Security Division; State of NY; NYC Police; City of Mobile, AL; Department of Justice Center for Domestic Preparedness; FBI; Wisconsin Office of Emergency Management; DOD; Indiana Office of State Fire Marshall; Jefferson County, MO

Manufacturer
Kappler Safety Group
70 Grimes Drive
Guntersville, AL 35976
http://www.kappler.com
POC: Kendra Barclay
256–505–4000 (Tel)
256–582–1163 (Fax)
email: kbarclay@kappler.com

Manufacturer Type Domestic

Developer Kappler Protective Apparel and Fabrics

Source http://www.kappler.com

Certification None

Operational Parameters

Chemical Warfare (CW) Agents Protected Against None

Biological Warfare (BW) Agents Protected Against Not applicable

Toxic Industrial (TIMs) Protected Against Carbon disulfide, sulfuric acid, ammonia, chlorine, hydrogen chloride, and ethylene oxide

Duration of Protection >480 min

Recommended Use(s) Kappler recommends that CPF 4 be used in chemical applications where the risk of coming in contact with chemical is high splash

Physical Parameters

Sizes Available S through 3XL

Weight 9 lb per case, 6 per case

Package Size and Volume Not specified

Power Requirements Not applicable

Material Type Multi-layer barrier film laminated to a 2.3 oz polypropylene substrate

Construction Type	Strapped seams
Color	Green
Logistical Parameters	
Ease of Use	Some instruction required
Consumables	Not applicable
Maintenance Requirements	Suits should be stored in a cool dry area away from direct sunlight. Level A garments should have a visual test and be pressure tested according to the ASTM F1052 Air Pressure Test Method upon arrival from manufacture, annually and/or after each use and a quick reinspection before each use .
Shelf Life	Under proper storage conditions there is no evidence to indicate that the System CPF® film composite fabrics lose their protective characteristics or physical properties over time. This conclusion is based on the comparative testing of "aged" and new Responder® fabric. Chemical suits contain components made from various polymer or rubber materials for which there is no specific shelf life data currently available. Based on the physical condition of the suit, it is recommended that downgrading suits to "training use only" be considered when they no longer pass the visual inspection and/or pressure test.
Transportability	Not applicable
Operational Limitations	Temperature service range: -85 °F to 200 °F
Environmental Conditions	Protective clothing is used under a variety of conditions. Garments can be exposed to a range of ambient temperatures as well as variations in the temperatures of the challenge chemical. The temperature service range for Responder and CPF 1–4 fabrics was established by performing tests at high and low temperatures. The high temperature was established by ASTM D751, "Test Methods for Coated Fabrics," using the high temperature blocking test. In this test, the sample fabric material is subjected to the predetermined temperature for a period of time while the fabric is placed in contact with itself. The test was run at 200 °F and the fabrics were considered nonblocking at that temperature. The low temperature was established by ASTM D 2136 "Standard Test Method for Coated Fabrics—Low Temperature Bend Test". This test subjects the fabric material to a predetermined low temperature for a period of time while the material is flexed in a 60° bend. The sample is then examined visually for signs of cracking or other damage. The test was run at -85 °F and the fabrics showed no signs of damage.
Unit Cost	Contact customer service for pricing
Maintenance Cost	Product is designed for limited use
Warranty	It is the responsibility of the user to select suits which are appropriate for each intended use and which meet all health standards. Kappler is available for consultation on any proposed use. Purchaser and all suit users shall promptly notify Kappler of any claim, whether based on contract, negligence, strict liability or otherwise. The sole and exclusive remedy of the purchaser and all users and the limit of liability of Kappler for any and all losses, injuries or damages resulting from use of a Kappler product shall be the refund of the purchase price or the replacement or repair of product found to be defective within 90 d after the product is delivered. In no event shall Kappler be liable for any special, incidental or consequential damages, whether in contract or in tort, arising out of

any warranties, representations, instructions or defects from any cause in connection with the Kappler products, or the sale thereof. The purchaser and the users are deemed to have accepted the terms of this limitation of warranty and liability, which terms may not be varied by any verbal or written agreement. Purchaser and all users are responsible for inspection and proper care of this product as described in the manual and are responsible for all loss or damage from use or handling which results from conditions beyond the control of the manufacturer.

Don/Doff Information	See instruction manual for instructions on donning and doffing
Use/Reuse	It is completely up to the discretion of the person wearing the suit. Kappler considers CPF 4 a limited use suit and reuse is based on both an evaluation of the physical state of the garment and also the level and type of chemical exposure.
Launderability	See instruction manual for instructions on donning and doffing
Accessories	Additional accessories that may be purchased include pressure test kit, chemtape, kooljacket, Tingley HazMat boot, and decontamination shower

Special Requirements

Training Requirements	Some instruction required
Training Available	Training video available, Suit Smart CD
Manuals Available	Instruction manual available
Surveillance Testing Requirements	Visual Inspections upon receipt from manufacturer, after each use, and before the next use
Support Equipment	Appropriate respiratory equipment
Testing Information	ASTM D751 Test Battery
Applicable Regulations	OSHA 1910.132 and OSHA 1910.120
Health Hazards	Not applicable
Communications Interface Capability	Not applicable
EOD Compatibility	Not applicable

General

Name — *Kappler CPF 4 Hood*
Item # 38

Picture Not Available

Technology — Multi-layer barrier film composite laminated to a high strength 2.3 oz polypropylene substrate

Stock Number — 4T651

Protection Type — Percutaneous

Equipment Category — Hood in waist length dickie style; PVC face shield, velcro closures on both sides, elastic at shoulders

Availability — In stock

Current User(s) — REC's Customers: EPA; Department of State Consequence Management and Diplomatic Security Division; State of NY; NYC Police; City of Mobile, AL; Department of Justice Center for Domestic Preparedness; FBI; Wisconsin Office of Emergency Management; DOD; and Indiana Office of State Fire Marshall; Jefferson County, MO.

Manufacturer —
Kappler Safety Group
70 Grimes Drive
Guntersville, AL 35976
http://www.kappler.com
POC: Kendra Barclay
256–505–4000 (Tel)
256–582–1163 (Fax)
email: kbarclay@kappler.com

Manufacturer Type — Domestic

Developer — Kappler Protective Apparel and Fabrics

Source — http://www.kappler.com

Certification — None

Operational Parameters

Chemical Warfare (CW) Agents Protected Against — None

Biological Warfare (BW) Agents Protected Against — Not applicable

Toxic Industrial (TIMs) Protected Against — Carbon disulfide, sulfuric acid, ammonia, chlorine, hydrogen chloride, and ethylene oxide

Duration of Protection — >480 min

Recommended Use(s) — Kappler recommends that CPF 4 be used in chemical applications where the risk of coming in contact with chemical is high splash

Physical Parameters

Sizes Available — S through 3XL

Weight — 10 lb, 6 per case

Package Size and Volume — Not specified

Power Requirements — Not applicable

Material Type — Multi-layer barrier film laminated to a 2.3 oz polypropylene substrate

Construction Type	Strapped seams
Color	Green
Logistical Parameters	
Ease of Use	Some instruction required
Consumables	Not applicable
Maintenance Requirements	Suits should be stored in a cool dry area away from direct sunlight. Level A garments should have a visual test and be pressure tested according to the ASTM F1052 Air Pressure Test Method upon arrival from manufacture, annually and/or after each use and a quick reinspection before each use.
Shelf Life	Under proper storage conditions there is no evidence to indicate that the System CPF® film composite fabrics lose their protective characteristics or physical properties over time. This conclusion is based on the comparative testing of "aged" and new Responder® fabric. Chemical suits contain components made from various polymer or rubber materials for which there is no specific shelf life data currently available. Based on the physical condition of the suit, it is recommended that downgrading suits to "training use only" be considered when they no longer pass the visual inspection and/or pressure test.
Transportability	Not applicable
Operational Limitations	Temperature service range: -85 °F to 200 °F
Environmental Conditions	Protective clothing is used under a variety of conditions. Garments can be exposed to a range of ambient temperatures as well as variations in the temperatures of the challenge chemical. The temperature service range for Responder and CPF 1–4 fabrics was established by performing tests at high and low temperatures. The high temperature was established by ASTM D751, "Test Methods for Coated Fabrics," using the high temperature blocking test. In this test, the sample fabric material is subjected to the predetermined temperature for a period of time while the fabric is placed in contact with itself. The test was run at 200 °F and the fabrics were considered nonblocking at that temperature. The low temperature was established by ASTM D 2136, "Standard Test Method for Coated Fabrics—Low Temperature Bend Test." This test subjects the fabric material to a predetermined low temperature for a period of time while the material is flexed in a 60° bend. The sample is then examined visually for signs of cracking or other damage. The test was run at -85 °F and the fabrics showed no signs of damage.
Unit Cost	Contact customer service for pricing
Maintenance Cost	Product is designed for limited use
Warranty	It is the responsibility of the user to select suits which are appropriate for each intended use and which meet all health standards. Kappler is available for consultation on any proposed use. Purchaser and all suit users shall promptly notify Kappler of any claim, whether based on contract, negligence, strict liability or otherwise. The sole and exclusive remedy of the purchaser and all users and the limit of liability of Kappler for any and all losses, injuries or damages resulting from use of a Kappler product shall be the refund of the purchase price or the replacement or repair of product found to be defective within 90 d after the product is delivered. In no event shall Kappler be liable for any special, incidental or consequential damages, whether in contract or in tort, arising out of

any warranties, representations, instructions or defects from any cause in connection with the Kappler products, or the sale thereof. The purchaser and the users are deemed to have accepted the terms of this limitation of warranty and liability, which terms may not be varied by any verbal or written agreement. Purchaser and all users are responsible for inspection and proper care of this product as described in the manual and are responsible for all loss or damage from use or handling which results from conditions beyond the control of the manufacturer.

Don/Doff Information	See instruction manual for instructions on donning and doffing
Use/Reuse	It is completely up to the discretion of the person wearing the suit. Kappler considers CPF 4 a limited use suit and reuse is based on both an evaluation of the physical state of the garment and also the level and type of chemical exposure.
Launderability	See instruction manual for instructions on donning and doffing
Accessories	Additional accessories that may be purchased include chemtape, kooljacket, Tingley HazMat boot, and decontamination shower

Special Requirements

Training Requirements	Some instruction required
Training Available	Training video available, Suit Smart CD
Manuals Available	Instruction manual available
Surveillance Testing Requirements	Visual Inspections upon receipt from manufacturer, after each use, and before the next use
Support Equipment	Appropriate respiratory equipment
Testing Information	ASTM D751 Test Battery
Applicable Regulations	OSHA 1910.132 and OSHA 1910.120
Health Hazards	Not applicable
Communications Interface Capability	Not applicable
EOD Compatibility	Not applicable

General

Name — *Kappler CPF 4 Jacket*

Item # 39

Picture Not Available

Technology — Multi-layer barrier film composite laminated to a high strength 2.3 oz polypropylene substrate

Stock Number — 4T670

Protection Type — Percutaneous

Equipment Category — Jacket—zipper front with double storm flap, mandarin collar, elastic wrists

Availability — In stock

Current User(s) — REC's Customers: EPA; Department of State Consequence Management and Diplomatic Security Division; State of NY; NYC Police; City of Mobile, AL; Department of Justice Center for Domestic Preparedness; FBI; Wisconsin Office of Emergency Management; DOD; and Indiana Office of State Fire Marshall; Jefferson County, MO.

Manufacturer —
Kappler Safety Group
70 Grimes Drive
Guntersville, AL 35976
http://www.kappler.com
POC: Kendra Barclay
256–505–4000 (Tel)
256–582–1163 (Fax)
email: kbarclay@kappler.com

Manufacturer Type — Domestic

Developer — Kappler Protective Apparel and Fabrics

Source — http://www.kappler.com

Certification — None

Operational Parameters

Chemical Warfare (CW) Agents Protected Against — None

Biological Warfare (BW) Agents Protected Against — Not applicable

Toxic Industrial (TIMs) Protected Against — Carbon disulfide, sulfuric acid, ammonia, chlorine, hydrogen chloride, and ethylene oxide

Duration of Protection — >480 min

Recommended Use(s) — Kappler recommends that CPF 4 be used in chemical applications where the risk of coming in contact with chemical is high splash

Physical Parameters

Sizes Available — S through 3XL

Weight — 10 lb/4.5kg, 6 per case

Package Size and Volume — Not specified

Power Requirements — Not applicable

Material Type	Multi-layer barrier film laminated to a 2.3 oz polypropylene substrate
Construction Type	Strapped seams
Color	Green
Logistical Parameters	
Ease of Use	Some instruction required
Consumables	Not applicable
Maintenance Requirements	Suits should be stored in a cool dry area away from direct sunlight. Level A garments should have a visual test and be pressure tested according to the ASTM F1052 Air Pressure Test Method upon arrival from manufacture, annually and/or after each use and a quick reinspection before each use.
Shelf Life	Under proper storage conditions there is no evidence to indicate that the System CPF® film composite fabrics lose their protective characteristics or physical properties over time. This conclusion is based on the comparative testing of "aged" and new Responder® fabric. Chemical suits contain components made from various polymer or rubber materials for which there is no specific shelf life data currently available. Based on the physical condition of the suit, it is recommended that downgrading suits to "training use only" be considered when they no longer pass the visual inspection and/or pressure test.
Transportability	Not applicable
Operational Limitations	Temperature service range: -85 °F to 200 °F
Environmental Conditions	Protective clothing is used under a variety of conditions. Garments can be exposed to a range of ambient temperatures as well as variations in the temperatures of the challenge chemical. The temperature service range for Responder and CPF 1–4 fabrics was established by performing tests at high and low temperatures. The high temperature was established by ASTM D751, "Test Methods for Coated Fabrics," using the high temperature blocking test. In this test, the sample fabric material is subjected to the predetermined temperature for a period of time while the fabric is placed in contact with itself. The test was run at 200° and the fabrics were considered nonblocking at that temperature. The low temperature was established by ASTM D 2136, "Standard Test Method for Coated Fabrics—Low Temperature Bend Test." This test subjects the fabric material to a predetermined low temperature for a period of time while the material is flexed in a 60 ° bend. The sample is then examined visually for signs of cracking or other damage. The test was run at -85 °F and the fabrics showed no signs of damage.
Unit Cost	Contact customer service for pricing
Maintenance Cost	Product is designed for limited use

Warranty	It is the responsibility of the user to select suits which are appropriate for each intended use and which meet all health standards. Kappler is available for consultation on any proposed use. Purchaser and all suit users shall promptly notify Kappler of any claim, whether based on contract, negligence, strict liability or otherwise. The sole and exclusive remedy of the purchaser and all users and the limit of liability of Kappler for any and all losses, injuries or damages resulting from use of a Kappler product shall be the refund of the purchase price or the replacement or repair of product found to be defective within 90 d after the product is delivered. In no event shall Kappler be liable for any special, incidental or consequential damages, whether in contract or in tort, arising out of any warranties, representations, instructions or defects from any cause in connection with the Kappler products, or the sale thereof. The purchaser and the users are deemed to have accepted the terms of this limitation of warranty and liability, which terms may not be varied by any verbal or written agreement. Purchaser and all users are responsible for inspection and proper care of this product as described in the manual and are responsible for all loss or damage from use or handling which results from conditions beyond the control of the manufacturer.
Don/Doff Information	See attached instruction manual for instructions on donning and doffing
Use/Reuse	It is completely up to the discretion of the person wearing the suit. Kappler considers CPF 4 a limited use suit and reuse is based on both an evaluation of the physical state of the garment and also the level and type of chemical exposure.
Launderability	See attached instruction manual for instructions on donning and doffing
Accessories	Additional accessories that may be purchased include pressure test kit, chemtape, kooljacket, Tingley HazMat boot, and decontamination shower

Special Requirements

Training Requirements	Some instruction required
Training Available	Training video available, Suit Smart CD
Manuals Available	Instruction manual available
Surveillance Testing Requirements	Visual Inspections upon receipt from manufacturer, after each use, and before the next use
Support Equipment	Appropriate respiratory equipment
Testing Information	ASTM D751 Test Battery
Applicable Regulations	OSHA 1910.132 and OSHA 1910.120
Health Hazards	Not applicable
Communications Interface Capability	Not applicable
EOD Compatibility	Not applicable

General

Name — *Lakeland Tychem® 10000 Level B Jacket*

Item # 40

Technology — Selectively permeable

Stock Number — 10260

Protection Type — Percutaneous

Equipment Category — Jacket, (hood with drawstring, zipper front, double storm flap with velcro, and elastic wrists)

Availability — 4 wk to 5 wk ARO

Current User(s) — Government organizations, municipal HazMat teams, fire departments, international HazMat/military organizations, and industry

Manufacturer — Lakeland Industries, Inc.
202 Pride Lane, SW
Decatur, AL 35602
POC: Carl Brown (Technical Product Specialist)
POC: Steve McCully (Product Manager)
800–645–9291 (Tel)
256–350–3011 (Fax)
Internet: http://www.lakeland.com

Manufacturer Type — Domestic

Developer — Lakeland Industries

Source — http://www.lakeland.com

Certification — Not applicable

Operational Parameters

Chemical Warfare (CW) Agents Protected Against — Nerve agents (GA, GB, GD, and VX); blister agents (HD and L). For specific test results, call the DuPont Protective Apparel Fax-on-Demand Service at 800–558–9329 and request Document 595.

Biological Warfare (BW) Agents Protected Against — Protects against all biological toxins and pathogens

Toxic Industrial (TIMs) Protected Against — Excellent protection against a wide variety of TIMs

Duration of Protection — Minimum of 8 h

Recommended Use(s) — Tactical operations, HazMat teams, chemical/biological testing, training, and warfare environments

Physical Parameters

Sizes Available — S through 5X

Weight — 12 pounds per case, 6 in a case

Package Size and Volume	Not specified
Power Requirements	None
Material Type	Garment is selectively permeable
Construction Type	Seam sewn and the heat-sealed with tape
Color	Lime-green

Logistical Parameters

Ease of Use	Garment poses no major mobility of flexibility problems from wearer compared to other Level B CPC
Consumables	None
Maintenance Requirements	Not specified
Shelf Life	After 5 yr, recommended to use only for training
Transportability	No support equipment required for transportation
Operational Limitations	Off the shelf cooling systems are available. Operational limitations to be decided by safety manager.
Environmental Conditions	Operational temperature range of Tychem 10000 material is -25 °F to 225 °F
Unit Cost	Cost to be determined by distributors
Maintenance Cost	Not applicable
Warranty	90 d
Don/Doff Information	Not specified
Use/Reuse	Limited use
Launderability	Suits are not launderable
Accessories	None

Special Requirements

Training Requirements	Not specified
Training Available	Available through regional sales representation
Manuals Available	User Manual and Permeation Guide available
Surveillance Testing Requirements	Visually inspect prior to use for holes or tears
Support Equipment	None
Testing Information	Not specified
Applicable Regulations	None
Health Hazards	None
Communications Interface Capability	Option is available
EOD Compatibility	Yes

General

Name — *Lakeland Tychem® 10000 Level B Overalls*
Item # 41

Technology — Selectively permeable
Stock Number — 10320
Protection Type — Percutaneous
Equipment Category — Overalls, bib pants with adjustable suspenders, and hemmed cuffs
Availability — 4 wk to 5 wk ARO
Current User(s) — Government organizations, municipal HazMat teams, fire departments, international HazMat/military organizations, and industry
Manufacturer — Lakeland Industries, Inc.
202 Pride Lane, SW
Decatur, AL 35602
POC: Carl Brown (Technical Product Specialist)
POC: Steve McCully (Product Manager)
800–645–9291 (Tel)
256–350–3011 (Fax)
Internet: http://www.lakeland.com
Manufacturer Type — Domestic
Developer — Lakeland Industries
Source — http://www.lakeland.com
Certification — Not applicable

Operational Parameters

Chemical Warfare (CW) Agents Protected Against — Nerve agents (GA, GB, GD, and VX); blister agents (HD and L). For specific test results, call the DuPont Protective Apparel Fax-on-Demand Service at 800–558–9329 and request Document 595.

Biological Warfare (BW) Agents Protected Against — Protects against all biological toxins and pathogens

Toxic Industrial (TIMs) Protected Against — Excellent protection against a wide variety of TIMs

Duration of Protection — Minimum of 8 h

Recommended Use(s) — Tactical operations, HazMat teams, chemical/biological testing, training, and warfare environments

Physical Parameters

Sizes Available — Small through 5X
Weight — 12 lb per case, 6 in a case
Package Size and Volume — Not specified

Power Requirements	None
Material Type	Garment is selectively permeable
Construction Type	Seam sewn and the heat-sealed with tape
Color	Lime-green
Logistical Parameters	
Ease of Use	Garment poses no major mobility of flexibility problems from wearer compared to other Level B CPC
Consumables	None
Maintenance Requirements	Not specified
Shelf Life	After 5 yr, recommended to use only for training
Transportability	No support equipment required for transportation
Operational Limitations	Off the shelf cooling systems are available. Operational limitations to be decided by safety manager.
Environmental Conditions	Operational temperature range of Tychem 10000 material is -25 °F to 225 °F
Unit Cost	Cost to be determined by distributors
Maintenance Cost	Not applicable
Warranty	90 d
Don/Doff Information	Not specified
Use/Reuse	Limited use
Launderability	Suits are not launderable
Accessories	None
Special Requirements	
Training Requirements	Not specified
Training Available	Available through regional sales representation
Manuals Available	User Manual and Permeation Guide available
Surveillance Testing Requirements	Visually inspect prior to use for holes or tears
Support Equipment	None
Testing Information	Not specified
Applicable Regulations	None
Health Hazards	None
Communications Interface Capability	Option is available
EOD Compatibility	Yes

General

Name *Lakeland Tychem® 10000 Level B Hood*
Item # 42

Technology	Selectively permeable
Stock Number	10716
Protection Type	Percutaneous
Equipment Category	Hood, bib style, 20 mil PVC faceshield, and velcro straps
Availability	4 wk to 5 wk ARO
Current User(s)	Government organizations, municipal HazMat teams, fire departments, international HazMat/military organizations, and industry
Manufacturer	Lakeland Industries, Inc. 202 Pride Lane, SW Decatur, AL 35602 POC: Carl Brown (Technical Product Specialist) POC: Steve McCully (Product Manager) 800–645–9291 (Tel) 256–350–3011 (Fax) Internet: http://www.lakeland.com
Manufacturer Type	Domestic
Developer	Lakeland Industries
Source	http://www.lakeland.com
Certification	Not applicable

Operational Parameters

Chemical Warfare (CW) Agents Protected Against	Nerve agents (GA, GB, GD, and VX); blister agents (HD and L). For specific test results, call the DuPont Protective Apparel Fax-on-Demand Service at 800–558–9329 and request Document 595.
Biological Warfare (BW) Agents Protected Against	Protects against all biological toxins and pathogens
Toxic Industrial (TIMs) Protected Against	Excellent protection against a wide variety of TIMs
Duration of Protection	Minimum of 8 h
Recommended Use(s)	Tactical operations, HazMat teams, chemical/biological testing, training, and warfare environments

Physical Parameters

Sizes Available	S through 5X
Weight	12 lb per case, 6 in a case

Package Size and Volume	Not specified
Power Requirements	None
Material Type	Garment is selectively permeable
Construction Type	Seam sewn and the heat-sealed with tape
Color	Lime-green

Logistical Parameters

Ease of Use	Garment poses no major mobility of flexibility problems from wearer compared to other Level B CPC
Consumables	None
Maintenance Requirements	Not specified
Shelf Life	After 5 yr, recommended to use only for training
Transportability	No support equipment required for transportation
Operational Limitations	Off the shelf cooling systems are available. Operational limitations to be decided by safety manager.
Environmental Conditions	Operational temperature range of Tychem 10000 material is -25 °F to 225 °F
Unit Cost	Cost to be determined by distributors
Maintenance Cost	Not applicable
Warranty	90 d
Don/Doff Information	Not specified
Use/Reuse	Limited use
Launderability	Suits are not launderable
Accessories	None

Special Requirements

Training Requirements	Not specified
Training Available	Available through regional sales representation
Manuals Available	User Manual and Permeation Guide available
Surveillance Testing Requirements	Visually inspect prior to use for holes or tears
Support Equipment	None
Testing Information	Not specified
Applicable Regulations	None
Health Hazards	None
Communications Interface Capability	Option is available
EOD Compatibility	Yes

General

Name — *Lakeland Tychem® 10000 Level B Apron*
Item # 43

Picture Not Available

Technology — Selectively permeable
Stock Number — 10730
Protection Type — Percutaneous
Equipment Category — Apron, long sleeves, elastic wrists, velcro straps at neck, and tie in back
Availability — 4 wk to 5 wk ARO
Current User(s) — Government organizations, municipal HazMat teams, fire departments, international HazMat/military organizations, and industry
Manufacturer — Lakeland Industries, Inc.
202 Pride Lane, SW
Decatur, AL 35602
POC: Carl Brown (Technical Product Specialist)
POC: Steve McCully (Product Manager)
800–645–9291 (Tel)
256–350–3011 (Fax)
Internet: http://www.lakeland.com
Manufacturer Type — Domestic
Developer — Lakeland Industries
Source — http://www.lakeland.com
Certification — Not applicable

Operational Parameters

Chemical Warfare (CW) Agents Protected Against — Nerve agents (GA, GB, GD, and VX); blister agents (HD and L). For specific test results, call the DuPont Protective Apparel Fax-on-Demand Service at 800–558–9329 and request Document 595.

Biological Warfare (BW) Agents Protected Against — Protects against all biological toxins and pathogens

Toxic Industrial (TIMs) Protected Against — Excellent protection against a wide variety of TIMs

Duration of Protection — Minimum of 8 h

Recommended Use(s) — Tactical operations, HazMat teams, chemical/biological testing, training, and warfare environments

Physical Parameters

Sizes Available — S through 5X
Weight — 12 lb per case, 12 in a case
Package Size and Volume — Not specified
Power Requirements — None
Material Type — Garment is selectively permeable
Construction Type — Seam sewn and the heat-sealed with tape
Color — Lime-green

Logistical Parameters

Ease of Use	Garment poses no major mobility of flexibility problems from wearer compared to other Level B CPC
Consumables	None
Maintenance Requirements	Not specified
Shelf Life	After 5 yr, recommended to use only for training
Transportability	No support equipment required for transportation
Operational Limitations	Off the shelf cooling systems are available. Operational limitations to be decided by safety manager.
Environmental Conditions	Operational temperature range of Tychem 10000 material is -25 °F to 225 °F
Unit Cost	Cost to be determined by distributors
Maintenance Cost	Not applicable
Warranty	90 d
Don/Doff Information	Not specified
Use/Reuse	Limited use
Launderability	Suits are not launderable
Accessories	None

Special Requirements

Training Requirements	Not specified
Training Available	Available through regional sales representation
Manuals Available	User Manual and Permeation Guide available
Surveillance Testing Requirements	Visually inspect prior to use for holes or tears
Support Equipment	None
Testing Information	Not specified
Applicable Regulations	None
Health Hazards	None
Communications Interface Capability	Option is available
EOD Compatibility	Yes

General

Name *Lakeland Tyvek® QC Level B Jacket*

Item # 44

Technology Selectively permeable

Stock Number 70250

Protection Type Percutaneous

Equipment Category Jacket, collar, double storm flap with velcro, zipper, and elastic wrists

Availability 4 wk to 5 wk ARO

Current User(s) Government organizations, municipal HazMat teams, fire departments, international HazMat/military organizations, industry

Manufacturer Lakeland Industries, Inc.
202 Pride Lane, SW
Decatur, AL 35602
POC: Carl Brown (Technical Product Specialist)
POC: Steve McCully (Product Manager)
800–645–9291 (Tel)
256–350–3011 (Fax)
Internet: http://www.lakeland.com

Manufacturer Type Domestic

Developer Lakeland Industries

Source http://www.lakeland.com

Certification Not applicable

Operational Parameters

Chemical Warfare (CW) Agents Protected Against Not tested

Biological Warfare (BW) Agents Protected Against Not specified

Toxic Industrial (TIMs) Protected Against Many inorganic acids, bases, and other liquid chemicals such as pesticides. Questions call Lakeland Customer Service at 800–645–9291.

Duration of Protection For specific TIMs data, contact Lakeland Customer Service at 800–645–9291

Recommended Use(s) Tactical operations, HazMat teams, chemical/biological testing, training, and warfare environments

Physical Parameters

Sizes Available S to 5X

Weight 6 lb per case, 6 in a case

Package Size and Volume Not specified

Power Requirements	None
Material Type	Garment is selectively permeable
Construction Type	Sealed seam
Color	Yellow or grey
Logistical Parameters	
Ease of Use	Garment poses no major mobility of flexibility problems from wearer compared to other Level B CPC
Consumables	None
Maintenance Requirements	Not specified
Shelf Life	After 5 yr, recommended to use only for training
Transportability	No support equipment required for transportation
Operational Limitations	Off the shelf cooling systems are available. Operational limitations to be decided by safety manager.
Environmental Conditions	Designed to be worn in common outdoor conditions
Unit Cost	Cost to be determined by distributors
Maintenance Cost	Not applicable
Warranty	90 d
Don/Doff Information	Not specified
Use/Reuse	Limited use
Launderability	Suits are not launderable
Accessories	None
Special Requirements	
Training Requirements	None
Training Available	Available through regional sales representation
Manuals Available	User Manual and Permeation Guide available
Surveillance Testing Requirements	Visually inspect prior to use for holes or tears
Support Equipment	None
Testing Information	Not specified
Applicable Regulations	None
Health Hazards	None
Communications Interface Capability	Option is available
EOD Compatibility	Yes

General

Name — *Lakeland Tyvek® QC Level B Pants*
Item # 45

Technology — Selectively permeable
Stock Number — 70300
Protection Type — Percutaneous
Equipment Category — Pants, elastic waist, and hemmed cuffs
Availability — 4 wk to 5 wk ARO
Current User(s) — Government organizations, municipal HazMat teams, fire departments, international HazMat/military organizations, and industry
Manufacturer — Lakeland Industries, Inc.
202 Pride Lane, SW
Decatur, AL 35602
POC: Carl Brown (Technical Product Specialist)
POC: Steve McCully (Product Manager)
800–645–9291 (Tel)
256–350–3011 (Fax)
Internet: http://www.lakeland.com
Manufacturer Type — Domestic
Developer — Lakeland Industries
Source — http://www.lakeland.com
Certification — Not applicable

Operational Parameters

Chemical Warfare (CW) Agents Protected Against — Not tested
Biological Warfare (BW) Agents Protected Against — Not specified
Toxic Industrial (TIMs) Protected Against — Many inorganic acids, bases, and other liquid chemicals such as pesticides. Questions call Lakeland Customer Service at 800–645–9291.
Duration of Protection — For specific TIMs data, contact Lakeland Customer Service at 800–645–9291
Recommended Use(s) — Tactical operations, HazMat teams, chemical/biological testing, training, and warfare environments

Physical Parameters

Sizes Available — S to 5X
Weight — 6 lb per case, 6 in a case

Package Size and Volume	Not specified
Power Requirements	None
Material Type	Garment is selectively permeable
Construction Type	Sealed seam
Color	Yellow or grey

Logistical Parameters

Ease of Use	Garment poses no major mobility of flexibility problems from wearer compared to other Level B CPC
Consumables	None
Maintenance Requirements	Not specified
Shelf Life	After 5 yr, recommended to use only for training
Transportability	No support equipment required for transportation
Operational Limitations	Off the shelf cooling systems are available. Operational limitations to be decided by safety manager.
Environmental Conditions	Designed to be worn in common outdoor conditions
Unit Cost	Cost to be determined by distributors
Maintenance Cost	Not applicable
Warranty	90 d
Don/Doff Information	Not specified
Use/Reuse	Limited use
Launderability	Suits are not launderable
Accessories	None

Special Requirements

Training Requirements	None
Training Available	Available through regional sales representation
Manuals Available	User Manual and Permeation Guide available
Surveillance Testing Requirements	Visually inspect prior to use for holes or tears
Support Equipment	None
Testing Information	Not specified
Applicable Regulations	None
Health Hazards	None
Communications Interface Capability	Option is available
EOD Compatibility	Yes

General

Name *Lakeland Tyvek® QC Level B Hood*
Item # 46

Technology Selectively permeable
Stock Number 70710
Protection Type Percutaneous
Equipment Category Hood, bell shape, and elastic face pullover
Availability 4 wk to 5 wk ARO
Current User(s) Government organizations, municipal HazMat teams, fire departments, international HazMat/military organizations, and industry
Manufacturer Lakeland Industries, Inc.
202 Pride Lane, SW
Decatur, AL 35602
POC: Carl Brown (Technical Product Specialist)
POC: Steve McCully (Product Manager)
800–645–9291 (Tel)
256–350–3011 (Fax)
Internet: http://www.lakeland.com
Manufacturer Type Domestic
Developer Lakeland Industries
Source http://www.lakeland.com
Certification Not applicable

Operational Parameters

Chemical Warfare (CW) Agents Protected Against Not tested
Biological Warfare (BW) Agents Protected Against Not specified
Toxic Industrial (TIMs) Protected Against Many inorganic acids, bases, and other liquid chemicals such as pesticides. Questions call Lakeland Customer Service at 800–645–9291.
Duration of Protection For specific TIMs data, contact Lakeland Customer Service at 800–645–9291
Recommended Use(s) Tactical operations, HazMat teams, chemical/biological testing, training, and warfare environments

Physical Parameters

Sizes Available 1 size
Weight 6 lb per case, 12 in a case

Package Size and Volume	Not specified
Power Requirements	None
Material Type	Garment is selectively permeable
Construction Type	Sealed seam
Color	Yellow or Grey

Logistical Parameters

Ease of Use	Garment poses no major mobility of flexibility problems from wearer compared to other Level B CPC
Consumables	None
Maintenance Requirements	Not specified
Shelf Life	After 5 yr, recommended to use only for training
Transportability	No support equipment required for transportation
Operational Limitations	Off the shelf cooling systems are available. Operational limitations to be decided by safety manager.
Environmental Conditions	Designed to be worn in common outdoor conditions
Unit Cost	Cost to be determined by distributors
Maintenance Cost	Not applicable
Warranty	90 d
Don/Doff Information	Not specified
Use/Reuse	Limited use
Launderability	Suits are not launderable
Accessories	None

Special Requirements

Training Requirements	None
Training Available	Available through regional sales representation
Manuals Available	User Manual and Permeation Guide available
Surveillance Testing Requirements	Visually inspect prior to use for holes or tears
Support Equipment	None
Testing Information	Not specified
Applicable Regulations	None
Health Hazards	None
Communications Interface Capability	Option is available
EOD Compatibility	Yes

General

Name *Lakeland Tyvek® QC Level B Sleeves*

Item # 47

Technology	Selectively permeable
Stock Number	70765
Protection Type	Percutaneous
Equipment Category	Sleeves (18 in length, elastic ends)
Availability	4 wk to 5 wk ARO
Current User(s)	Government organizations, municipal HazMat teams, fire departments, international HazMat/military organizations, and industry
Manufacturer	Lakeland Industries, Inc. 202 Pride Lane, SW Decatur, AL 35602 POC: Carl Brown (Technical Product Specialist) POC: Steve McCully (Product Manager) 800-645-9291 (Tel) 256-350-3011 (Fax) Internet: http://www.lakeland.com
Manufacturer Type	Domestic
Developer	Lakeland Industries
Source	http://www.lakeland.com
Certification	Not applicable

Operational Parameters

Chemical Warfare (CW) Agents Protected Against	Not tested
Biological Warfare (BW) Agents Protected Against	Not specified
Toxic Industrial (TIMs) Protected Against	Many inorganic acids, bases, and other liquid chemicals such as pesticides. Questions call Lakeland Customer Service at 800-645-9291.
Duration of Protection	For specific TIMs data, contact Lakeland Customer Service at 800-645-9291
Recommended Use(s)	Tactical operations, HazMat teams, chemical/biological testing, training, and warfare environments

Physical Parameters

Sizes Available	18 in length
Weight	6 lb per case, 12 in a case

Package Size and Volume	Not specified
Power Requirements	None
Material Type	Garment is selectively permeable
Construction Type	Sealed seam
Color	Yellow or grey

Logistical Parameters

Ease of Use	Garment poses no major mobility of flexibility problems from wearer compared to other Level B CPC
Consumables	None
Maintenance Requirements	Not specified
Shelf Life	After 5 yr, recommended to use only for training
Transportability	No support equipment required for transportation
Operational Limitations	Off the shelf cooling systems are available. Operational limitations to be decided by safety manager.
Environmental Conditions	Designed to be worn in common outdoor conditions
Unit Cost	Cost to be determined by distributors
Maintenance Cost	Not applicable
Warranty	90 d
Don/Doff Information	Not specified
Use/Reuse	Limited use
Launderability	Suits are not launderable
Accessories	None

Special Requirements

Training Requirements	None
Training Available	Available through regional sales representation
Manuals Available	User Manual and Permeation Guide available
Surveillance Testing Requirements	Visually inspect prior to use for holes or tears
Support Equipment	None
Testing Information	Not specified
Applicable Regulations	None
Health Hazards	None
Communications Interface Capability	Option is available
EOD Compatibility	Yes

General

Name — *Lakeland Tychem® SL Level B Hood*

Item # 48

Technology	Selectively permeable
Stock Number	72710
Protection Type	Percutaneous
Equipment Category	Hood, pullover, bell shape, and elastic face
Availability	4 wk to 5 wk ARO
Current User(s)	Government organizations, municipal HazMat teams, fire departments, international HazMat/military organizations, and industry
Manufacturer	Lakeland Industries, Inc. 202 Pride Lane, SW Decatur, AL 35602 POC: Carl Brown (Technical Product Specialist) POC: Steve McCully (Product Manager) 800–645–9291 (Tel) 256–350–3011 (Fax) Internet: http://www.lakeland.com
Manufacturer Type	Domestic
Developer	Lakeland Industries
Source	http://www.lakeland.com
Certification	Not applicable

Operational Parameters

Chemical Warfare (CW) Agents Protected Against	Nerve agents (GB and VX); blister agents (HD and L). Questions call Lakeland Customer Service at 800–645–9291.
Biological Warfare (BW) Agents Protected Against	Not specified
Toxic Industrial (TIMs) Protected Against	A broad range of liquid chemicals. Questions call Lakeland Customer Service at 800–645–9291.
Duration of Protection	Fabric test data: Average breakthrough time VX: Greater than 12 h at 10 g/m^2 GB and L: Greater than 6 h at 10 g/m^2 D: Greater than 3 h at 10 g/m^2 Questions call Lakeland Customer Service at 800–645–9291
Recommended Use(s)	Tactical operations, HazMat teams, chemical/biological testing, training, and warfare environments

Physical Parameters

Sizes Available	One size
Weight	6 lb per case, 12 in a case
Package Size and Volume	Not specified
Power Requirements	None
Material Type	Garment is selectively permeable
Construction Type	Seam sewn and the heat-sealed with tape
Color	White

Logistical Parameters

Ease of Use	Garment poses no major mobility of flexibility problems from wearer compared to other Level B CPC
Consumables	None
Maintenance Requirements	Not specified
Shelf Life	After 5 yr, recommended to use only for training
Transportability	No support equipment required for transportation
Operational Limitations	Off the shelf cooling systems are available. Operational limitations to be decided by safety manager.
Environmental Conditions	Designed to be worn in common outdoor conditions
Unit Cost	Cost to be determined by distributors
Maintenance Cost	Not applicable
Warranty	90 d
Don/Doff Information	Not specified
Use/Reuse	Limited use
Launderability	Suits are not launderable
Accessories	None

Special Requirements

Training Requirements	Not specified
Training Available	Available through regional sales representation
Manuals Available	User Manual and Permeation Guide available
Surveillance Testing Requirements	Visually inspect prior to use for holes or tears
Support Equipment	None
Testing Information	Not specified
Applicable Regulations	None
Health Hazards	None
Communications Interface Capability	Option is available
EOD Compatibility	Yes

General

Name *Lakeland Tychem® SL Level B Hood*
Item # 49

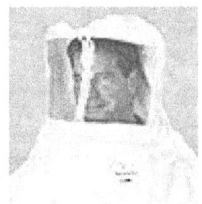

Technology	Selectively permeable
Stock Number	72712
Protection Type	Percutaneous
Equipment Category	Hood, bell shape, 20 mil PVC face shield, and velcro straps under arm
Availability	4 wk to 5 wk ARO
Current User(s)	Government organizations, municipal HazMat teams, fire departments, international HazMat/military organizations, and industry
Manufacturer	Lakeland Industries, Inc. 202 Pride Lane, SW Decatur, AL 35602 POC: Carl Brown (Technical Product Specialist) POC: Steve McCully (Product Manager) 800–645–9291 (Tel) 256–350–3011 (Fax) Internet: http://www.lakeland.com
Manufacturer Type	Domestic
Developer	Lakeland Industries
Source	http://www.lakeland.com
Certification	Not applicable

Operational Parameters

Chemical Warfare (CW) Agents Protected Against	Nerve agents (GB and VX); blister agents (HD and L). Questions call Lakeland Customer Service at 800–645–9291.
Biological Warfare (BW) Agents Protected Against	Not specified
Toxic Industrial (TIMs) Protected Against	A broad range of liquid chemicals. Questions call Lakeland Customer Service at 800–645–9291.
Duration of Protection	Fabric test data: Average breakthrough time VX: Greater than 12 h at 10 g/m^2 GB and L: Greater than 6 h at 10 g/m^2 D: Greater than 3 h at 10 g/m^2 Questions call Lakeland Customer Service at 800–645–9291
Recommended Use(s)	Tactical operations, HazMat teams, chemical/biological testing, training, and warfare environments.

Physical Parameters

Sizes Available	1 size
Weight	6 lb per case, 6 in a case
Package Size and Volume	Not specified
Power Requirements	None
Material Type	Garment is selectively permeable
Construction Type	Seam sewn and the heat-sealed with tape
Color	White

Logistical Parameters

Ease of Use	Garment poses no major mobility of flexibility problems from wearer compared to other Level B CPC
Consumables	None
Maintenance Requirements	Not specified
Shelf Life	After 5 yr, recommended to use only for training
Transportability	No support equipment required for transportation
Operational Limitations	Off the shelf cooling systems are available. Operational limitations to be decided by safety manager.
Environmental Conditions	Designed to be worn in common outdoor conditions
Unit Cost	Cost to be determined by distributors
Maintenance Cost	Not applicable
Warranty	90 d
Don/Doff Information	Not specified
Use/Reuse	Limited use
Launderability	Suits are not launderable
Accessories	None

Special Requirements

Training Requirements	Not specified
Training Available	Available through regional sales representation
Manuals Available	User Manual and Permeation Guide available
Surveillance Testing Requirements	Visually inspect prior to use for holes or tears
Support Equipment	None
Testing Information	Not specified
Applicable Regulations	None
Health Hazards	None
Communications Interface Capability	Option is available
EOD Compatibility	Yes

General

Name — *Lakeland Tychem® SL Level B Apron*

Item # 50

Technology	Selectively permeable
Stock Number	72735
Protection Type	Percutaneous
Equipment Category	Apron, bib style, knee length, ties at neck, and waist
Availability	4 wk to 5 wk ARO
Current User(s)	Government organizations, municipal HazMat teams, fire departments, international HazMat/military organizations, and industry
Manufacturer	Lakeland Industries, Inc. 202 Pride Lane, SW Decatur, AL 35602 POC: Carl Brown (Technical Product Specialist) POC: Steve McCully (Product Manager) 800–645–9291 (Tel) 256–350–3011 (Fax) Internet: http://www.lakeland.com
Manufacturer Type	Domestic
Developer	Lakeland Industries
Source	http://www.lakeland.com
Certification	Not applicable

Operational Parameters

Chemical Warfare (CW) Agents Protected Against	Nerve agents (GB and VX); blister agents (HD and L). Questions call Lakeland Customer Service at 800–645–9291.
Biological Warfare (BW) Agents Protected Against	Not specified
Toxic Industrial (TIMs) Protected Against	A broad range of liquid chemicals. Questions call Lakeland Customer Service at 800–645–9291.
Duration of Protection	Fabric test data: Average breakthrough time VX: Greater than 12 h at 10 g/m^2 GB and L: Greater than 6 h at 10 g/m^2 D: Greater than 3 h at 10 g/m^2 Questions call Lakeland Customer Service at 800–645–9291
Recommended Use(s)	Tactical operations, HazMat teams, chemical/biological testing, training, and warfare environments

Physical Parameters

Sizes Available	1 size
Weight	8 lb per case, 12 in a case
Package Size and Volume	Not specified
Power Requirements	None
Material Type	Garment is selectively permeable
Construction Type	Seam sewn and the heat-sealed with tape
Color	White

Logistical Parameters

Ease of Use	Garment poses no major mobility of flexibility problems from wearer compared to other Level B CPC
Consumables	None
Maintenance Requirements	Not specified
Shelf Life	After 5 yr, recommended to use only for training
Transportability	No support equipment required for transportation
Operational Limitations	Off the shelf cooling systems are available. Operational limitations to be decided by safety manager.
Environmental Conditions	Designed to be worn in common outdoor conditions
Unit Cost	Cost to be determined by distributors
Maintenance Cost	Not applicable
Warranty	90 d
Don/Doff Information	Not specified
Use/Reuse	Limited use
Launderability	Suits are not launderable
Accessories	None

Special Requirements

Training Requirements	None
Training Available	Available through regional sales representation
Manuals Available	User Manual and Permeation Guide available
Surveillance Testing Requirements	Visually inspect prior to use for holes or tears
Support Equipment	None
Testing Information	Not specified
Applicable Regulations	None
Health Hazards	None
Communications Interface Capability	Option is available
EOD Compatibility	Yes

General

Name — *Lakeland Tychem® SL Level B Boots*

Item # 51

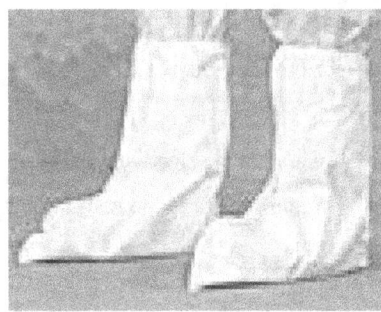

Technology	Selectively permeable
Stock Number	72740
Protection Type	Percutaneous
Equipment Category	Boots (elastic at top)
Availability	4 wk to 5 wk ARO
Current User(s)	Government organizations, municipal HazMat teams, fire departments, international HazMat/military organizations, and industry
Manufacturer	Lakeland Industries, Inc. 202 Pride Lane, SW Decatur, AL 35602 POC: Carl Brown (Technical Product Specialist) POC: Steve McCully (Product Manager) 800–645–9291 (Tel) 256–350–3011 (Fax) Internet: http://www.lakeland.com
Manufacturer Type	Domestic
Developer	Lakeland Industries
Source	http://www.lakeland.com
Certification	Not applicable

Operational Parameters

Chemical Warfare (CW) Agents Protected Against	Nerve agents (GB and VX); blister agents (HD and L). Questions call Lakeland Customer Service at 800–645–9291.
Biological Warfare (BW) Agents Protected Against	Not specified
Toxic Industrial (TIMs) Protected Against	A broad range of liquid chemicals. Questions call Lakeland Customer Service at 800–645–9291.
Duration of Protection	Fabric test data: Average breakthrough time VX: Greater than 12 h at 10 g/m^2 GB and L: Greater than 6 h at 10 g/m^2 D: Greater than 3 h at 10 g/m^2 Questions call Lakeland Customer Service at 800–645–9291
Recommended Use(s)	Tactical operations, HazMat teams, chemical/biological testing, training, and warfare environments

Physical Parameters

Sizes Available	1 size
Weight	7 lb per case, 12 in a case
Package Size and Volume	Not specified
Power Requirements	None
Material Type	Garment is selectively permeable
Construction Type	Seam sewn and the heat-sealed with tape
Color	White

Logistical Parameters

Ease of Use	Garment poses no major mobility of flexibility problems from wearer compared to other Level B CPC
Consumables	None
Maintenance Requirements	Not specified
Shelf Life	After 5 yr, recommended to use only for training
Transportability	No support equipment required for transportation
Operational Limitations	Off the shelf cooling systems are available. Operational limitations to be decided by safety manager.
Environmental Conditions	Designed to be worn in common outdoor conditions
Unit Cost	Cost to be determined by distributors
Maintenance Cost	Not applicable
Warranty	90 d
Don/Doff Information	Not specified
Use/Reuse	Limited use
Launderability	Suits are not launderable
Accessories	None

Special Requirements

Training Requirements	None
Training Available	Available through regional sales representation
Manuals Available	User Manual and Permeation Guide available
Surveillance Testing Requirements	Visually inspect prior to use for holes or tears
Support Equipment	None
Testing Information	Not specified
Applicable Regulations	None
Health Hazards	None
Communications Interface Capability	Option is available
EOD Compatibility	Yes

General
Name — *Lakeland Tychem® SL Level B Sleeves*
Item # 52

Technology — Selectively permeable
Stock Number — 72765
Protection Type — Percutaneous
Equipment Category — Sleeves (elastic ends, 18 in length)
Availability — 4 wk to 5 wk ARO
Current User(s) — Government organizations, municipal HazMat teams, fire departments, international HazMat/military organizations, and industry
Manufacturer — Lakeland Industries, Inc.
202 Pride Lane, SW
Decatur, AL 35602
POC: Carl Brown (Technical Product Specialist)
POC: Steve McCully (Product Manager)
800–645–9291 (Tel)
256–350–3011 (Fax)
Internet: http://www.lakeland.com

Manufacturer Type — Domestic
Developer — Lakeland Industries
Source — http://www.lakeland.com
Certification — Not applicable

Operational Parameters
Chemical Warfare (CW) Agents Protected Against — Nerve agents (GB and VX); blister agents (HD and L). Questions call Lakeland Customer Service at 800–645–9291.

Biological Warfare (BW) Agents Protected Against — Not specified

Toxic Industrial (TIMs) Protected Against — A broad range of liquid chemicals. Questions call Lakeland Customer Service at 800–645–9291.

Duration of Protection — Fabric test data: Average breakthrough time
VX: Greater than 12 h at 10 g/m^2
GB and L: Greater than 6 h at 10 g/m^2
D: Greater than 3 h at 10 g/m^2
Questions call Lakeland Customer Service at 800–645–9291

Recommended Use(s) — Tactical operations, HazMat teams, chemical/biological testing, training, and warfare environments

Physical Parameters

Sizes Available	18 in length
Weight	6 lb per case, 12 in a case
Package Size and Volume	Not specified
Power Requirements	None
Material Type	Garment is selectively permeable
Construction Type	Seam sewn and the heat-sealed with tape
Color	White

Logistical Parameters

Ease of Use	Garment poses no major mobility of flexibility problems from wearer compared to other Level B CPC
Consumables	None
Maintenance Requirements	Not specified
Shelf Life	After 5 yr, recommended to use only for training
Transportability	No support equipment required for transportation
Operational Limitations	Off the shelf cooling systems are available. Operational limitations to be decided by safety manager.
Environmental Conditions	Designed to be worn in common outdoor conditions
Unit Cost	Cost to be determined by distributors
Maintenance Cost	Not applicable
Warranty	90 d
Don/Doff Information	Not specified
Use/Reuse	Limited use
Launderability	Suits are not launderable
Accessories	None

Special Requirements

Training Requirements	None
Training Available	Available through regional sales representation
Manuals Available	User Manual and Permeation Guide available
Surveillance Testing Requirements	Visually inspect prior to use for holes or tears
Support Equipment	None
Testing Information	Not specified
Applicable Regulations	None
Health Hazards	None
Communications Interface Capability	Option is available
EOD Compatibility	Yes

General

Name — *Lakeland Tychem® 9400 Level B Jacket/Pants*

Item # 53

Technology — Selectively permeable

Stock Number — 94250—jacket
94300—pants

Protection Type — Percutaneous

Equipment Category — Jacket/pants; jacket with collar, elastic wrists, zipper closure with storm flaps; pants with elastic waist, and hemmed cuffs

Availability — 4 wk to 5 wk ARO

Current User(s) — Government organizations, municipal HazMat teams, fire departments, international HazMat/military organizations, and industry

Manufacturer — Lakeland Industries, Inc.
202 Pride Lane, SW
Decatur, AL 35602
POC: Carl Brown (Technical Product Specialist)
POC: Steve McCully (Product Manager)
800–645–9291 (Tel)
256–350–3011 (Fax)
Internet: http://www.lakeland.com

Manufacturer Type — Domestic

Developer — Lakeland Industries

Source — http://www.lakeland.com

Certification — Not applicable

Operational Parameters

Chemical Warfare (CW) Agents Protected Against — Nerve agents (GA, GB, GD, and VX); blister agents (HD and L)

Biological Warfare (BW) Agents Protected Against — Not specified

Toxic Industrial (TIMs) Protected Against — A broad range of TIMs. Contact Lakeland for further information.

Duration of Protection — Breakthrough time at minimum of 8 h, except ammonia at 45 min, dichloromethane at 391 min, and methanol at 150 min

Recommended Use(s) — Tactical operations, HazMat teams, chemical/biological testing, training, and warfare environments

Physical Parameters

Sizes Available	S through 5X
Weight	94250—8 lb per case, 6 in a case
	94300—6 lb per case, 6 in a case
Package Size and Volume	Not specified
Power Requirements	None
Material Type	Garment is selectively permeable
Construction Type	Seam sewn and the heat-sealed with tape
Color	Schoolbus yellow

Logistical Parameters

Ease of Use	Garment poses no major mobility or flexibility problems from wearer compared to other Level B CPC
Consumables	None
Maintenance Requirements	Not specified
Shelf Life	After 5 yr, recommended to use only for training
Transportability	No support equipment required for transportation
Operational Limitations	Off the shelf cooling systems are available. Operational limitations to be decided by safety manager.
Environmental Conditions	Designed to be worn in common outdoor conditions
Unit Cost	Cost to be determined by distributors
Maintenance Cost	Not applicable
Warranty	90 d
Don/Doff Information	Not specified
Use/Reuse	Limited use
Launderability	Suits are not launderable
Accessories	None

Special Requirements

Training Requirements	Not specified
Training Available	Available through regional sales representation
Manuals Available	User Manual and Permeation Guide available
Surveillance Testing Requirements	Visually inspect prior to use for holes or tears
Support Equipment	None
Testing Information	Not specified
Applicable Regulations	None
Health Hazards	None
Communications Interface Capability	Option is available
EOD Compatibility	Yes

General

Name
Item # 54

Lakeland Tychem® 9400 Level B Hood

Technology — Selectively permeable
Stock Number — 94710
Protection Type — Percutaneous
Equipment Category — Hood (pullover, bell shape, and elastic face)
Availability — 4 wk to 5 wk ARO
Current User(s) — Government organizations, municipal HazMat teams, fire departments, international HazMat/military organizations, and industry

Manufacturer —
Lakeland Industries, Inc.
202 Pride Lane, SW
Decatur, AL 35602
POC: Carl Brown (Technical Product Specialist)
POC: Steve McCully (Product Manager)
800–645–9291 (Tel)
256–350–3011 (Fax)
Internet: http://www.lakeland.com

Manufacturer Type — Domestic
Developer — Lakeland Industries
Source — http://www.lakeland.com
Certification — Not applicable

Operational Parameters

Chemical Warfare (CW) Agents Protected Against — Nerve agents (GA, GB, GD, and VX); blister agents (HD and L)

Biological Warfare (BW) Agents Protected Against — Not specified

Toxic Industrial (TIMs) Protected Against — A broad range of TIMs. Contact Lakeland for further information.

Duration of Protection — Breakthrough time at minimum of 8 h, except Ammonia at 45 min, Dichloromethane at 391 min, and Methanol at 150 min

Recommended Use(s) — Tactical operations, hazmat teams, chemical/biological testing, training, and warfare environments

Physical Parameters

Sizes Available — 1 size
Weight — 10 lb per case, 12 in a case

Package Size and Volume	Not specified
Power Requirements	None
Material Type	Garment is selectively permeable
Construction Type	Seam sewn and the heat-sealed with tape
Color	Schoolbus yellow

Logistical Parameters

Ease of Use	Garment poses no major mobility or flexibility problems from wearer compared to other Level B CPC
Consumables	None
Maintenance Requirements	Not specified
Shelf Life	After 5 yr, recommended to use only for training
Transportability	No support equipment required for transportation
Operational Limitations	Off the shelf cooling systems are available. Operational limitations to be decided by safety manager.
Environmental Conditions	Designed to be worn in common outdoor conditions
Unit Cost	Cost to be determined by distributors
Maintenance Cost	Not applicable
Warranty	90 d
Don/Doff Information	Not specified
Use/Reuse	Limited use
Launderability	Suits are not launderable
Accessories	None

Special Requirements

Training Requirements	None
Training Available	Available through regional sales representation
Manuals Available	User Manual and Permeation Guide available
Surveillance Testing Requirements	Visually inspect prior to use for holes or tears
Support Equipment	None
Testing Information	Not specified
Applicable Regulations	None
Health Hazards	None
Communications Interface Capability	Option is available
EOD Compatibility	Yes

General

Name — *Lakeland Tychem® 9400 Level B Hood*

Item # 55

Technology	Selectively permeable
Stock Number	94712
Protection Type	Percutaneous
Equipment Category	Hood, (bell shape, 20 mil PVC faceshield, and velcro straps under arm)
Availability	4 wk to 5 wk ARO
Current User(s)	Government organizations, municipal HazMat teams, fire departments, international HazMat/military organizations, and industry
Manufacturer	Lakeland Industries, Inc. 202 Pride Lane, SW Decatur, AL 35602 POC: Carl Brown (Technical Product Specialist) POC: Steve McCully (Product Manager) 800–645–9291 (Tel) 256–350–3011 (Fax) Internet: http://www.lakeland.com
Manufacturer Type	Domestic
Developer	Lakeland Industries
Source	http://www.lakeland.com
Certification	Not applicable

Operational Parameters

Chemical Warfare (CW) Agents Protected Against	Nerve agents (GA, GB, GD, and VX); blister agents (HD and L)
Biological Warfare (BW) Agents Protected Against	Not specified
Toxic Industrial (TIMs) Protected Against	A broad range of TIMs. Contact Lakeland for further information.
Duration of Protection	Breakthrough time at minimum of 8 h, except Ammonia at 45 min, Dichloromethane at 391 min, and Methanol at 150 min
Recommended Use(s)	Tactical operations, hazmat teams, chemical/biological testing, training, and warfare environments

Physical Parameters

Sizes Available	1 size
Weight	10 lb per case, 6 in a case

Package Size and Volume	Not specified
Power Requirements	None
Material Type	Garment is selectively permeable
Construction Type	Seam sewn and the heat-sealed with tape
Color	Schoolbus yellow

Logistical Parameters

Ease of Use	Garment poses no major mobility or flexibility problems from wearer compared to other Level B CPC
Consumables	None
Maintenance Requirements	Not specified
Shelf Life	After 5 yr, recommended to use only for training
Transportability	No support equipment required for transportation
Operational Limitations	Off the shelf cooling systems are available. Operational limitations to be decided by safety manager.
Environmental Conditions	Designed to be worn in common outdoor conditions
Unit Cost	Cost to be determined by distributors
Maintenance Cost	Not applicable
Warranty	90 d
Don/Doff Information	Not specified
Use/Reuse	Limited use
Launderability	Suits are not launderable
Accessories	None

Special Requirements

Training Requirements	None
Training Available	Available through regional sales representation
Manuals Available	User Manual and Permeation Guide available
Surveillance Testing Requirements	Visually inspect prior to use for holes or tears
Support Equipment	None
Testing Information	Not specified
Applicable Regulations	None
Health Hazards	None
Communications Interface Capability	Option is available
EOD Compatibility	Yes

General

Name — Lakeland Tychem® 9400 Level B Apron

Item # 56

Picture Not Available

Technology — Selectively permeable

Stock Number — 94735

Protection Type — Percutaneous

Equipment Category — Apron, (bib style, knee length, ties at neck, and waist)

Availability — 4 wk to 5 wk ARO

Current User(s) — Government organizations, municipal HazMat teams, fire departments, international HazMat/military organizations, and industry

Manufacturer — Lakeland Industries, Inc.
202 Pride Lane, SW
Decatur, AL 35602
POC: Carl Brown (Technical Product Specialist)
POC: Steve McCully (Product Manager)
800–645–9291 (Tel)
256–350–3011 (Fax)
Internet: http://www.lakeland.com

Manufacturer Type — Domestic

Developer — Lakeland Industries

Source — http://www.lakeland.com

Certification — Not applicable

Operational Parameters

Chemical Warfare (CW) Agents Protected Against — Nerve agents (GA, GB, GD, and VX); blister agents (HD and L)

Biological Warfare (BW) Agents Protected Against — Not specified

Toxic Industrial (TIMs) Protected Against — A broad range of TIMs. Contact Lakeland for further information.

Duration of Protection — Breakthrough time at minimum of 8 h, except Ammonia at 45 min, Dichloromethane at 391 min, and Methanol at 150 min

Recommended Use(s) — Tactical operations, hazmat teams, chemical/biological testing, training, and warfare environments

Physical Parameters

Sizes Available — 1 size

Weight — 10 lb per case, 12 in a case

Package Size and Volume — Not specified

Power Requirements — None

Material Type — Garment is selectively permeable

Construction Type — Seam sewn and the heat-sealed with tape

Color — Schoolbus yellow

Logistical Parameters

Ease of Use	Garment poses no major mobility or flexibility problems from wearer compared to other Level B CPC
Consumables	None
Maintenance Requirements	Not specified
Shelf Life	After 5 yr, recommended to use only for training
Transportability	No support equipment required for transportation
Operational Limitations	Off the shelf cooling systems are available. Operational limitations to be decided by safety manager.
Environmental Conditions	Designed to be worn in common outdoor conditions
Unit Cost	Cost to be determined by distributors
Maintenance Cost	Not applicable
Warranty	90 d
Don/Doff Information	Not specified
Use/Reuse	Limited use
Launderability	Suits are not launderable
Accessories	None

Special Requirements

Training Requirements	None
Training Available	Available through regional sales representation
Manuals Available	User Manual and Permeation Guide available
Surveillance Testing Requirements	Visually inspect prior to use for holes or tears
Support Equipment	None
Testing Information	Not specified
Applicable Regulations	None
Health Hazards	None
Communications Interface Capability	Option is available
EOD Compatibility	Yes

General
Name *Lakeland Tychem® 9400 Level B Sleeves*
Item # 57

Technology Selectively permeable
Stock Number 94765
Protection Type Percutaneous
Equipment Category Sleeves, (elastic ends)
Availability 4 wk to 5 wk ARO
Current User(s) Government organizations, municipal HazMat teams, fire departments, international HazMat/military organizations, and industry
Manufacturer Lakeland Industries, Inc.
202 Pride Lane, SW
Decatur, AL 35602
POC: Carl Brown (Technical Product Specialist)
POC: Steve McCully (Product Manager)
800–645–9291 (Tel)
256–350–3011 (Fax)
Internet: http://www.lakeland.com
Manufacturer Type Domestic
Developer Lakeland Industries
Source http://www.lakeland.com
Certification Not applicable

Operational Parameters
Chemical Warfare (CW) Agents Protected Against Nerve agents (GA, GB, GD, and VX); blister agents (HD and L)
Biological Warfare (BW) Agents Protected Against Not specified
Toxic Industrial (TIMs) Protected Against A broad range of TIMs. Contact Lakeland for further information.
Duration of Protection Breakthrough time at minimum of 8 h, except Ammonia at 45 min, Dichloromethane at 391 min, and Methanol at 150 min
Recommended Use(s) Tactical operations, hazmat teams, chemical/biological testing, training, and warfare environments

Physical Parameters
Sizes Available 18 in length
Weight 9 lb per case, 12 in a case

Package Size and Volume	Not specified
Power Requirements	None
Material Type	Garment is selectively permeable
Construction Type	Seam sewn and the heat-sealed with tape
Color	Schoolbus yellow

Logistical Parameters

Ease of Use	Garment poses no major mobility or flexibility problems from wearer compared to other Level B CPC
Consumables	None
Maintenance Requirements	Not specified
Shelf Life	After 5 yr, recommended to use only for training
Transportability	No support equipment required for transportation
Operational Limitations	Off the shelf cooling systems are available. Operational limitations to be decided by safety manager.
Environmental Conditions	Designed to be worn in common outdoor conditions
Unit Cost	Cost to be determined by distributors
Maintenance Cost	Not applicable
Warranty	90 d
Don/Doff Information	Not specified
Use/Reuse	Limited use
Launderability	Suits are not launderable
Accessories	None

Special Requirements

Training Requirements	None
Training Available	Available through regional sales representation
Manuals Available	User Manual and Permeation Guide available
Surveillance Testing Requirements	Visually inspect prior to use for holes or tears
Support Equipment	None
Testing Information	Not specified
Applicable Regulations	None
Health Hazards	None
Communications Interface Capability	Option is available
EOD Compatibility	Yes

General

Name	*Lakeland Tychem® 9400 Level B Boot Covers*
Item # 58	
Technology	Selectively permeable
Stock Number	94740
Protection Type	Percutaneous
Equipment Category	Boot covers (elastic at top)
Availability	4 wk to 5 wk ARO
Current User(s)	Government organizations, municipal HazMat teams, fire departments, international HazMat/military organizations, and industry
Manufacturer	Lakeland Industries, Inc. 202 Pride Lane, SW Decatur, AL 35602 POC: Carl Brown (Technical Product Specialist) POC: Steve McCully (Product Manager) 800–645–9291 (Tel) 256–350–3011 (Fax) Internet: http://www.lakeland.com
Manufacturer Type	Domestic
Developer	Lakeland Industries
Source	http://www.lakeland.com
Certification	Not applicable

Operational Parameters

Chemical Warfare (CW) Agents Protected Against	Nerve agents (GA, GB, GD, and VX); blister agents (HD and L)
Biological Warfare (BW) Agents Protected Against	Not specified
Toxic Industrial (TIMs) Protected Against	A broad range of TIMs. Contact Lakeland for further information..
Duration of Protection	Breakthrough time at minimum of 8 h, except ammonia at 45 min, dichloromethane at 391 min, and methanol at 150 min
Recommended Use(s)	Tactical operations, hazmat teams, chemical/biological testing, training, and warfare environments

Physical Parameters

Sizes Available	1 size
Weight	9 lb per case, 12 in a case

Package Size and Volume	Not specified
Power Requirements	None
Material Type	Garment is selectively permeable
Construction Type	Seam sewn and the heat-sealed with tape
Color	School Bus yellow

Logistical Parameters

Ease of Use	Garment poses no major mobility or flexibility problems from wearer compared to other Level B CPC
Consumables	None
Maintenance Requirements	Not specified
Shelf Life	After 5 yr, recommended to use only for training
Transportability	No support equipment required for transportation
Operational Limitations	Off the shelf cooling systems are available. Operational limitations to be decided by safety manager.
Environmental Conditions	Designed to be worn in common outdoor conditions
Unit Cost	Cost to be determined by distributors
Maintenance Cost	Not applicable
Warranty	90 d
Don/Doff Information	Not specified
Use/Reuse	Limited use
Launderability	Suits are not launderable
Accessories	None

Special Requirements

Training Requirements	None
Training Available	Available through regional sales representation
Manuals Available	User Manual and Permeation Guide available
Surveillance Testing Requirements	Visually inspect prior to use for holes or tears
Support Equipment	None
Testing Information	Not specified
Applicable Regulations	None
Health Hazards	None
Communications Interface Capability	Option is available
EOD Compatibility	Yes

General

Name *Chemical Protective Undergarment (CPU)*

Item # 59

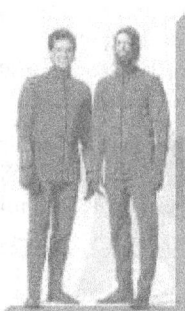

Technology LANX is a durable composite fabric containing polymerically encapsulated carbon for the adsorption of chemical warfare agents. The overgarment also features a shell fabric with flame resistant or nonflame resistant characteristics.

Stock Number Undershirt: 8415-01-363-8692 thru 8700 (last 4 indicates size)
Drawers: 8415-01-363-8683 thru 8691 (last 4 indicates size)
Large sizes of shirts and drawers available if required

Protection Type Percutaneous—Protects against CB agents

Equipment Category CPU consists of a shirt and drawers as well as accessories such as all fabric glove liners, boot liners, and balaclavas. Shirts are available with hoods upon request.

Availability Leadtime depends on order volume. All CPUs custom made to order.

Current User(s) Current users include the U.S. Special Forces, U.S. Technical Escort Unit, 4th WMD Civilian Support Team, Washington State Patrol, Seattle Police Department, St. Paul Police Department, St. Louis Police Department, DeMil Contractors, and the Royal Canadian Mounted Police (RCMP). Law enforcement applications include SWAT teams, bomb squads, narcotics units and security details. HazMat responders utilize the CPU as a backup level of protection in the event of a breach in their nonpermeable or fully encapsulated protective outer apparel. The CPU provides flexibility to the breadth of the first response community as the basis of a chemical/biological protective system.

Manufacturer LANX Fabric Systems
220 GBC Drive
Newark, DE 19702
POC: Randall D. Lofland
302–451–3060 (Tel)
302–451–0208 (Fax)
e-mail: randall.lofland@xymid.com

Manufacturer Type Domestic

Developer DuPont developed the LANX technology. LANX Fabric Systems has exclusive rights to manufacture and market the product.

Source LANX Fabric Systems

Certification All CPU's meet the chemical agent protective requirements of Military Specification MIL–U–44435. The only undergarment to qualify during JSLIST testing.

Operational Parameters

Chemical Warfare (CW) Distilled mustard (HD), soman (GD), thickened soman (TGD), Lewisite (L), VX, and other lower order agents such as sarin

Agents Protected Against
Biological Warfare (BW) Agents Protected Against

The CPU inherently protects against BW agents as the particulate size of a BW agent is larger than that of a CW agent making it easier to adsorb than CW agents.

Toxic Industrial (TIMs) Protected Against

Untested as of January 31, 2000, for TIMs application

Duration of Protection

The CPU has been tested and proven to provide 24 h of protection in a contaminated environment. Significantly reduces heat stress on user as a result of air permeable technology.

Recommended Use(s)

LANX recommends a systems approach to the CPU. An end user can successfully maintain protection from CB agents in addition to other threats by adding other types of protective apparel deemed appropriate to the threat, thus providing excellent protection from liquid, vapor, and aerosol threats. Examples of these systems include: Body armor and bomb suits worn over the CPU for agencies such as law enforcement. When worn beneath the body armor or bomb suit, the chemical protective integrity of the protective apparel stands a better chance of remaining in tact versus CPO in the event of a shooting, stabbing, or explosion. Tactical Units wear their duty uniform or tactical coverall with the CPU for better mobility and reduced heat stress during periods of heavy physical exertion while maintaining protection against CB threats HazMat or other responders utilize the CPU as a backup to a fully encapsulated (Level A) suit, or, as in the case of the U.S. Technical Escort Unit, with a Tyvek Suit to form a Level B ensemble. The US Military wears the CPU with the BDU and when coupled with the appropriate respiratory protection, assumes MOPP IV. Security details wear the CPU beneath duty uniforms or civilian clothing to establish a covert protective posture that does not alarm the public or alert the terrorist.

Physical Parameters

Sizes Available

Shirt: (chest) 32 thru 54
Drawers: (waist) 26 thru 48
Gloves: S, M, L, and XL
Boot liners: S, M, L, and XL

Weight

Weighs less than 3 lb per suit

Package Size and Volume

The CPU is vacuum packed and occupies approximately 1 ft^3 of space

Power Requirements

None

Material Type

Air permeable, sorptive technology made with polymerically encapsulated activated carbon

Construction Type

Seams not liquid proof

Color

Charcoal gray

Logistical Parameters

Ease of Use

Very easy to use, similar to putting on long underwear. Air permeable technology significantly reduces heat stress allowing the user to work exponentially longer than nonpermeable technologies.

Consumables

Not specified

Maintenance Requirements

Store in dry place, standard indoor warehouse conditions

Shelf Life

The ultimate shelf life of the CPU has yet to be determined. The technology is 10 yr old and shows no signs of degradation during annual testing. The US Military currently assesses the shelf life to be 12 yr.

Transportability	May be transported easily whether in a backpack, garment bag, tote bag, or even hand carried
Operational Limitations	The CPU provides excellent CB agent protection. Additional liquid and splash protection may come from a duty uniform, tyvek suit, fully encapsulated liquid barrier suit or other type of overgarment or shell fabric.
Environmental Conditions	The CPU works well in most climates. Due care should be taken to keep the CPU in a bag when not in use. The CPU's air permeable nature allows for the transportation of sweat away from the body, significantly reducing heat stress.
Unit Cost	Call for a quotation at 302-451-3060 POC: Randall D. Lofland
Maintenance Cost	None if stored properly
Warranty	The CPU is manufactured to Military Pattern PD 97-04 and meets the Chemical Protective requirements of Military Specification MIL-U-44435
Don/Doff Information	The CPU is easy to don and doff. One man may don and doff his own CPU under normal circumstances. Some agencies require a two man doffing procedure following contamination. Check your agency protocol.
Use/Reuse	The CPU may be reused after wearing and laundering. After contamination with CW agent, current military doctrine dictates disposing of the garment properly.
Launderability	Yes—The CPU is launderable up to 10 launderings if uncontaminated. If contaminated to agent, dispose of IAW procedures.
Accessories	The CPU has accessories such as all fabric glove liners, boot liners, balaclavas, and a shirt option with a hood

Special Requirements

Training Requirements	Minimal training required (< 20 min). Contaminated CPU doffing procedures may vary. Check local protocols
Training Available	Introductory training is available upon request.. Advanced training is based upon agency protocol and should be developed at the local level
Manuals Available	Care, use, and storage information is available if needed
Surveillance Testing Requirements	The manufacturer performs CCL4 testing annually prior to distribution to end users. The end user should visually inspect the CPU at regularly scheduled intervals.
Support Equipment	Not applicable
Testing Information	The most recent testing of the LANX CPU was performed using AVLAG Test Operating Procedure (TOP) 8-2-501. See JSLIST (MIL-U-44435).
Applicable Regulations	The CPU is governed by the International Traffic and Arms Regulations (ITAR)
Health Hazards	MSDSs are on file. No indication of health hazards present.
Communications Interface Capability	Not applicable
EOD Compatibility	Works well with a bomb squad application. CPUs are part of an ordnance application with Med-Eng bomb suits available for EOD applications through: Med-Eng Systems, Inc. 2400 St. Laurent Boulevard Ottawa, Ontario, Canada K1G 6C4 610-739-9646 (Tel)

General

Name — *Escape Jacket C/92F with optional Escape Hood*
Item # 60

Technology — Jacket is constructed from a 70 um 5 ply PE-EVAL film
Stock Number — C/92F
Protection Type — Percutaneous
Equipment Category — Plastic jacket with sealed sleeved ends. An integrated hood has a half mask assembled to the hood. An escape hood is available as an option.
Availability — Commercial
Current User(s) — Civilian or Military
Manufacturer —
New Pac Safety AB
P.O. Box 174
S–566 23 Habo
Sweden
+46 36 411 39 (Tel)
+46 36 410 31 (Fax)
e-mail: info@newpac.se

Manufacturer Type — Foreign
Developer — New Pac Safety AB
Source —
Sales: INDEF Services Intl.
14847 Lee Highway
Amissville, VA 20106–0089
540–937–7327 (Tel)
540–937–7328 (Fax)
e-mail: indefsteve@msn.com

Certification — Not specified

Operational Parameters

Chemical Warfare (CW) Agents Protected Against — NBC
Biological Warfare (BW) Agents Protected Against — Not specified
Toxic Industrial (TIMs) Protected Against — Most hazardous chemicals
Duration of Protection — The film provides chemical protection for more than 8 h
Recommended Use(s) — Personal NBC safe escape outfit

Physical Parameters

Sizes Available	Not specified
Weight	Lightweight
Package Size and Volume	Comes packed into a small textile bag
Power Requirements	Not applicable
Material Type	Jacket is constructed from a 70 um 5 ply PE-EVAL film
Construction Type	A thin plastic jacket with tightly sealed sleeve ends. The integrated hood has half mask assembled to the hood. The hood has a clear front for sufficient see through, and jacket has a waist seal.
Color	Military green

Logistical Parameters

Ease of Use	Not specified
Consumables	None
Maintenance Requirements	Not specified
Shelf Life	Not specified
Transportability	Not applicable
Operational Limitations	Not specified
Environmental Conditions	Not specified
Unit Cost	Not specified
Maintenance Cost	Not specified
Warranty	Not specified
Don/Doff Information	Not specified
Use/Reuse	Not specified
Launderability	Not specified
Accessories	Not specified

Special Requirements

Training Requirements	Not specified
Training Available	Not specified
Manuals Available	Not specified
Surveillance Testing Requirements	Not specified
Support Equipment	An Escape Hood C/92F is also available as an option
Testing Information	Not specified
Applicable Regulations	Not specified
Health Hazards	Not specified
Communications Interface Capability	Not specified
EOD Compatibility	Not specified

General

Name   *PONCHO NP/60*

Item # 61

Technology   Constructed from a 50 μm to 60 μm thick, rectangular shaped polyethylene film, containing no protective PA barrier

Stock Number   NATO Stock No: 8415 25 148 4799

Protection Type   Percutaneous

Equipment Category   Poncho - Designed to protect an ordinary textile/charcoal combat suit and to be worn before an expected warfare attack of C-drops falling from a height

Availability   Commercial

Current User(s)   Military

Manufacturer   New Pac Safety AB
P.O. Box 174
S-566 23 Habo
Sweden
+46 36 411 39 (Tel)
+46 36 410 31 (Fax)
e-mail: info@newpac.se

Manufacturer Type   Foreign

Developer   New Pac Safety AB

Source   Sales: INDEF Services Intl.
14847 Lee Highway
Amissville, VA 20106-0089
540-937-7327 (Tel)
540-937-7328 (Fax)
e-mail: indefsteve@msn.com

Certification   Not specified

Operational Parameters

Chemical Warfare (CW) Agents Protected Against   NBC

Biological Warfare (BW) Agents Protected Against   Not specified

Toxic Industrial (TIMs) Protected Against   Most hazardous chemicals

Duration of Protection   The film provides full protection against liquid warfare agents for at least 30 min

Recommended Use(s)   Military

Physical Parameters

Sizes Available	Not specified
Weight	Lightweight
Package Size and Volume	Not specified
Power Requirements	Not applicable
Material Type	Constructed from a 50 μm to 60 μm thick, rectangular shaped polyethylene film, containing no protective PA barrier
Construction Type	Rectangular shaped poncho. In the center of the poncho is an extended hood section with an elastic opening fitting tightly to the mask. The helmet may be worn inside the hood.
Color	Military green

Logistical Parameters

Ease of Use	Not specified
Consumables	None
Maintenance Requirements	Not specified
Shelf Life	Not specified
Transportability	Not applicable
Operational Limitations	Not specified
Environmental Conditions	Not specified
Unit Cost	Not specified
Maintenance Cost	Not specified
Warranty	Not specified
Don/Doff Information	Not specified
Use/Reuse	Not specified
Launderability	Not specified
Accessories	Not specified

Special Requirements

Training Requirements	Not specified
Training Available	Not specified
Manuals Available	Not specified
Surveillance Testing Requirements	Not specified
Support Equipment	Not specified
Testing Information	Not specified
Applicable Regulations	Not specified
Health Hazards	Not specified
Communications Interface Capability	Not specified
EOD Compatibility	Not specified

General
Name — *North Silver Shield Gloves*
Item # 62

Technology — Made from Norfoil, a lightweight, flexible laminate which resists permeation and breakthrough of many toxic/hazardous chemicals

Stock Number — Not specified
Protection Type — Percutaneous
Equipment Category — Gloves
Availability — Not specified
Current User(s) — Not specified
Manufacturer — North
Manufacturer Type — Not specified
Developer — North
Source — Ralmike's Tool-A-Rama, Inc.
524 Lincoln Boulevard
Middlesex, NJ 08846
800–462–4243 (Tel)
800–472–5645 (Fax)
Certification — Not specified

Operational Parameters
Chemical Warfare (CW) Agents Protected Against — Not specified
Biological Warfare (BW) Agents Protected Against — Not specified
Toxic Industrial (TIMs) Protected Against — Many hazardous chemicals
Duration of Protection — Not specified
Recommended Use(s) — Chemical and petrochemical laboratories, spill cleanups, and many other applications

Physical Parameters
Sizes Available — M and L
Weight — Not specified
Package Size and Volume — Not specified
Power Requirements — None
Material Type — Made from Norfoil, a lightweight, flexible laminate which resists permeation and breakthrough of many toxic/hazardous chemicals

Construction Type	Not specified
Color	Silver-gray
Logistical Parameters	
Ease of Use	Not specified
Consumables	None
Maintenance Requirements	None
Shelf Life	Not specified
Transportability	Not applicable
Operational Limitations	Not specified
Environmental Conditions	Not specified
Unit Cost	Not specified
Maintenance Cost	Not specified
Warranty	Not specified
Don/Doff Information	Not specified
Use/Reuse	Not specified
Launderability	Not specified
Accessories	Not specified
Special Requirements	
Training Requirements	None
Training Available	None
Manuals Available	Not specified
Surveillance Testing Requirements	Not specified
Support Equipment	Not specified
Testing Information	Not specified
Applicable Regulations	Not specified
Health Hazards	Not specified
Communications Interface Capability	Not specified
EOD Compatibility	Not specified

General

Name — *Rocky Shoes and Boots*

Item # 63

Picture Not Available

Technology — Crosstech* footwear fabric, from W.L. Gore and Associates, is durably waterproof, and bloodborne pathogen and common chemical penetration resistant

Stock Number — Eliminator 8030, 8032, 8036, and 8132
ANSI Eliminator Steel toe 6032 and 6432 (Women's)

Protection Type — Percutaneous

Equipment Category — Shoes and boots with Crosstech

Availability — In production

Current User(s) — U.S. Army, Air Force, Coast Guard, Police, and EMS

Manufacturer — Rocky Shoes and Boots, Inc.
39 East Canal St.
Nelsonville, OH 45764
POC: Mike Mikulecky
903–489–3673 (Tel)

Manufacturer Type — Domestic

Developer — Rocky Shoes and Boots, In.
Crosstech by Gore-Tex

Source — Rocky Shoes and Boots, Inc.

Certification — NFPA 1999 (Rocky* styles using Crosstech*), Protective Clothing for Emergency Medical Operations (1992 edition), ASTM F 1671 (Standard Test Method for Resistance of Protective Clothing Materials to Penetration by Bloodborne Pathogens), ASTM F 903 (C) (Standard Test Method for Resistance of Protective Clothing Materials to Penetration by Liquids)

Operational Parameters

Chemical Warfare (CW) Agents Protected Against — Not specified

Biological Warfare (BW) Agents Protected Against — Protective to penetration by bloodborne pathogens

Toxic Industrial (TIMs) Protected Against — TIMs not specified

Duration of Protection — Not specified

Recommended Use(s) — Resistant to common chemicals including battery acid, gasoline, hydraulic fluid, swimming pool chemicals, and aqueous film form foam

Physical Parameters

Sizes Available — 5 through 10 (women)
7 through 15 (men)

Weight — Not specified

Package Size and Volume — Not specified

Power Requirements — Not applicable

Material Type	Rocky® Eliminator® 2: Padded collar and tongue for comfortable fit. Durable yet lightweight 1000 denier Cordura® nylon, Cambrelle® lining, Thinsulate® insulation, waterproof full grain leather, and thermoplastic toe box. Sole: Dual density polyurethane outsole, Axidyne® polymer impact cushion, steel shank, Texon® insole for support, Axidyne* polymer impact cushion on forepart, and toe areas.
Construction Type	Direct attach construction sole to upper; double-stitched, and sealed seams
Color	Not specified
Logistical Parameters	
Ease of Use	Not applicable
Consumables	Not applicable
Maintenance Requirements	Not applicable
Shelf Life	Not specified
Transportability	Not applicable
Operational Limitations	Designed using dual density blown urethane footbed to cushion and cradle the foot. Air perforations in forepart allow for air exchange—creating both a cushioning and cooling sensation.
Environmental Conditions	Not specified
Unit Cost	~ $90
Maintenance Cost	Not applicable
Warranty	Not specified
Don/Doff Information	Not specified
Use/Reuse	Can be reused
Launderability	Soap and water
Accessories	Not applicable
Special Requirements	
Training Requirements	Not applicable
Training Available	Not applicable
Manuals Available	Not applicable
Surveillance Testing Requirements	Not applicable
Support Equipment	Not applicable
Testing Information	NFPA 1999 (Rocky* styles using Crosstech*), Protective Clothing for Emergency Medical Operations (1992 edition), ASTM F 1671 (Standard Test Method for Resistance of Protective Clothing Materials to Penetration by Bloodborne Pathogens), ASTM F 903 (C) (Standard Test Method for Resistance of Protective Clothing Materials to Penetration by Liquids)
Applicable Regulations	Not applicable
Health Hazards	Not applicable
Communications Interface Capability	Not applicable
EOD Compatibility	Not specified

General
Name — *Servus HZT Hazmat Knee Boot*

Item # 64

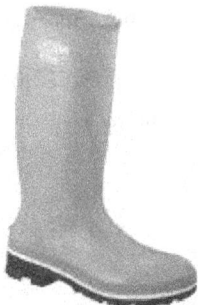

Technology	Safe-toe steel toe cap, puncture resistant steel toe midsole, foot form, and contour insole
Stock Number	Not specified
Protection Type	Percutaneous
Equipment Category	Boots
Availability	Not specified
Current User(s)	Not specified
Manufacturer	Servus Firefighter Footwear 1 Innovation Court Dayton, OH 45413 POC: Attn: Karen
Manufacturer Type	Not specified
Developer	Not specified
Source	http://www.servusfire.com email: shannont@totalfiregroup.com
Certification	NFPA 1991 Requirements

Operational Parameters

Chemical Warfare (CW) Agents Protected Against	Not specified
Biological Warfare (BW) Agents Protected Against	Not specified
Toxic Industrial (TIMs) Protected Against	Not specified
Duration of Protection	Not specified
Recommended Use(s)	HazMat

Physical Parameters

Sizes Available	Boot heights are proportioned to boot size
Weight	Not specified
Package Size and Volume	Not specified
Power Requirements	None
Material Type	Not specified
Construction Type	Safe-toe steel toe cap, puncture resistant steel toe midsole, foot form, and contour insole

Color	Green with black soles

Logistical Parameters

Ease of Use	Not specified
Consumables	None
Maintenance Requirements	None
Shelf Life	Not specified
Transportability	Not applicable
Operational Limitations	Not specified
Environmental Conditions	Not specified
Unit Cost	Not specified
Maintenance Cost	Not specified
Warranty	Not specified
Don/Doff Information	No assistance necessary
Use/Reuse	Not specified
Launderability	TDT self-cleaning outsole
Accessories	None

Special Requirements

Training Requirements	None
Training Available	None
Manuals Available	Not specified
Surveillance Testing Requirements	Not specified
Support Equipment	Not specified
Testing Information	Not specified
Applicable Regulations	Not specified
Health Hazards	Not specified
Communications Interface Capability	Not specified
EOD Compatibility	Not specified

General

Name	*Saratoga Chemical Protective Gloves*
Item # 65	
	Picture Not Available
Technology	Permeable Saratoga carbon sphere technology
Stock Number	TS CO–0326B
Protection Type	Percutaneous
Equipment Category	Gloves
Availability	Currently in production
Current User(s)	Local, State, and Federal law enforcement agencies
Manufacturer	Tex-Shield, Inc. 5206 Morrowick Rd. Charlotte, NC 28226 POC: Nona Fahl 704–341–3681 (Tel) 704–341–3468 (Fax)
Manufacturer Type	Domestic
Developer	Tex-Shield, Inc.
Source	Tex-Shield, Inc.
Certification	Meets chemical warfare agent protection requirements of MIL–C–29462 dated April 15, 1992

Operational Parameters

Chemical Warfare (CW) Agents Protected Against	All classes of chemical warfare agents when used as directed with chemical warfare protective mask, suit, and overboots or socks
Biological Warfare (BW) Agents Protected Against	Protects against biological warfare agents when used as directed with appropriate mask, suit, and overboots or socks
Toxic Industrial (TIMs) Protected Against	Not tested
Duration of Protection	Meet the requirements for protection from chemical warfare agents for up to 30 d wear, and 120 calendar days after initial usage or 24 h after contamination
Recommended Use(s)	Tactical operations

Physical Parameters

Sizes Available	S, M, L, and XL
Weight	Varies by size. Nominal weight < 0.5 lb/pair.
Package Size and Volume	Folded gloves in package fit into trouser pocket of Saratoga JSLIST or HAMMER suit
Power Requirements	None
Material Type	Saratoga permeable glove of activated carbon spheres on cotton knit. Leather palm provides additional chemical protection.
Construction Type	Seam sealing not required in Saratoga garments
Color	Green, black

Logistical Parameters

Ease of Use	Comfortable, breathable glove system for liquid and vapor chemical warfare contamination
Consumables	None
Maintenance Requirements	General inspection for holes and tears. Record wear use.
Shelf Life	10 yr
Transportability	Vacuum sealed, compact package
Operational Limitations	Durable glove system. Provides dexterity, comfort, and protection from chemical warfare agents. Glove should be protected by leather or appropriate work glove or overglove when necessary.
Environmental Conditions	No environmental usage limitations. Not effected by rain, fog, snow, salt, and water.
Unit Cost	$40 per system
Maintenance Cost	None
Warranty	Free of defects in material and workmanship for 1 yr
Don/Doff Information	Assistance is not required
Use/Reuse	Reusable
Launderability	Not machine launderable, spot clean
Accessories	Gloves may be purchased as package with Saratoga suits and socks

Special Requirements

Training Requirements	No special training required
Training Available	No special training required
Manuals Available	Instructions for use supplied with gloves
Surveillance Testing Requirements	No testing required. Inspection for tears and damage required.
Support Equipment	Chemical warfare protective mask, suits, and socks or overboots
Testing Information	Independent test data/certificate of compliance is available upon request.
Applicable Regulations	None
Health Hazards	None
Communications Interface Capability	Not applicable
EOD Compatibility	Interface with EOD CB protective suit

General

Name — *Saratoga Chemical Protective Socks*
Item # 66

Picture Not Available

Technology	Permeable Saratoga carbon sphere technology
Stock Number	TS CO–0356
Protection Type	Percutaneous
Equipment Category	Socks
Availability	Currently in production
Current User(s)	Local, State, and Federal law enforcement agencies
Manufacturer	Tex-Shield, Inc. 5206 Morrowick Rd. Charlotte, NC 28226 POC: Nona Fahl 704–341–3681 (Tel) 704–341–3468 (Fax)
Manufacturer Type	Domestic
Developer	Tex-Shield, Inc.
Source	Tex-Shield, Inc.
Certification	Meets system chemical tests requirements, Of PD 97–04

Operational Parameters

Chemical Warfare (CW) Agents Protected Against	All classes of chemical warfare agents when used as directed with chemical warfare protective mask, suit, and gloves
Biological Warfare (BW) Agents Protected Against	Protects against biological warfare agents when used as directed with appropriate mask, suit, and gloves
Toxic Industrial (TIMs) Protected Against	Not tested
Duration of Protection	Meet the requirements for protection from chemical warfare agents for up to 6 launderings, 30 d wear, 120 calendar days after initial usage or 24 h after contamination
Recommended Use(s)	Tactical operations, all law enforcement

Physical Parameters

Sizes Available	S, M, L, and XL
Weight	Varies by size. Nominal weight < 0.5 lb/pair.
Package Size and Volume	Folded socks in package fit into trouser pocket of Saratoga JSLIST or HAMMER suit
Power Requirements	None
Material Type	Saratoga permeable fabric of activated carbon spheres on cotton knit covered by lightweight, wicking, and thermoplastic knit. Not FR.
Construction Type	Seam sealing not required in Saratoga garments
Color	White, black

Logistical Parameters

Ease of Use	Lightweight, comfortable socks compatible with standard boots. No change in boot size is required.
Consumables	None
Maintenance Requirements	General garment inspection for holes and tears. Standard laundering. Record wear use and laundering.
Shelf Life	10 yr
Transportability	Vacuum sealed, compact package
Operational Limitations	Durable sock. Does not cause blisters when worn over standard socks with boots.
Environmental Conditions	No environmental usage limitations. Not effected by rain, fog, snow, salt, and water.
Unit Cost	$30 per system
Maintenance Cost	None
Warranty	Free of defects in material and workmanship for 1 yr
Don/Doff Information	Assistance is not required
Use/Reuse	Reusable and launderable
Launderability	Socks are launderable 6 times for hygienic purposes. Standard home laundering.
Accessories	Socks may be purchased as package with Saratoga suits and gloves

Special Requirements

Training Requirements	No special training required
Training Available	No special training required
Manuals Available	Instructions for use supplied with socks
Surveillance Testing Requirements	No testing required. Inspection for tears and damage required.
Support Equipment	Chemical warfare protective mask, suits, and gloves
Testing Information	Independent test data/certificate of compliance is available upon request.
Applicable Regulations	None
Health Hazards	None
Communications Interface Capability	Not applicable
EOD Compatibility	Interface with EOD CB protective suit

General

Name — *Saratoga Chemical Protective Undergarment*

Item # 67

Picture Not Available

Technology	Permeable Saratoga carbon sphere technology
Stock Number	TS U CO10356
Protection Type	Percutaneous
Equipment Category	Undergarment
Availability	Currently in production
Current User(s)	Local, State, and Federal law enforcement agencies
Manufacturer	Tex-Shield, Inc. 5206 Morrowick Rd. Charlotte, NC 28226 POC: Nona Fahl 704–341–3681 (Tel) 704–341–3468 (Fax)
Manufacturer Type	Domestic
Developer	Tex-Shield, Inc.
Source	Tex-Shield, Inc.
Certification	Meets vapor chemical warfare protection of MIL–C–29462

Operational Parameters

Chemical Warfare (CW) Agents Protected Against	Protects against all classes of vapor chemical warfare agents when used as directed with chemical warfare protective mask, boots or socks, and gloves. Liquid protection depends on outer clothing layer.
Biological Warfare (BW) Agents Protected Against	Protects against biological warfare agents when used as directed with appropriate mask, outer clothing, socks or boots, and gloves
Toxic Industrial (TIMs) Protected Against	Not tested
Duration of Protection	Meet the requirements for protection from chemical warfare agents for up to 6 launderings, 30 d wear, 120 calendar days after initial usage or 24 h after contamination. Liquid protection depends on outer clothing layer.
Recommended Use(s)	Tactical operations, intelligence, medical first responders

Physical Parameters

Sizes Available	S, M, L, and XL
Weight	Varies by size
Package Size and Volume	Nominal 10 in x 6 in x 3 in vacuum sealed package size for each piece
Power Requirements	None
Material Type	Saratoga permeable fabric of activated carbon spheres on cotton knit covered by lightweight, wicking, and thermoplastic knit. Not FR.
Construction Type	Seam sealing not required in Saratoga garments
Color	White, black

Logistical Parameters

Ease of Use	Lightweight, comfortable, compatible with other uniforms, and equipment
Consumables	None
Maintenance Requirements	General garment inspection for holes and tears. Standard laundering. Record wear use and laundering.
Shelf Life	10 yr
Transportability	Vacuum sealed, compact package
Operational Limitations	Durable undergarment. Liquid chemical protection depends on outer clothing layer.
Environmental Conditions	No environmental usage limitations. Not effected by rain, fog, snow, salt, and water.
Unit Cost	$180 per suit
Maintenance Cost	None
Warranty	Free of defects in material and workmanship for 1 yr
Don/Doff Information	Assistance is not required
Use/Reuse	Reusable and launderable
Launderability	Launderable 6 times for hygienic purposes. Standard home or industrial laundering.
Accessories	Undergarments may be purchased as package with Saratoga socks and gloves

Special Requirements

Training Requirements	No special training required
Training Available	No special training required
Manuals Available	Instructions for use included with garment
Surveillance Testing Requirements	No testing required. Inspection for tears and damage required.
Support Equipment	Chemical warfare protective mask, outer clothing, socks or overboots and gloves
Testing Information	Independent test data/certificate of compliance is available upon request.
Applicable Regulations	None
Health Hazards	None
Communications Interface Capability	Not applicable
EOD Compatibility	Interface with EOD protective suit

General

Name — *Tingley Hazproof Overboot*

Item # 68

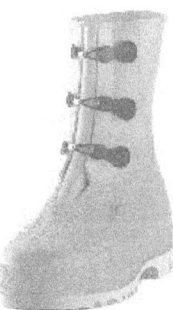

Technology — Fire retardant PVC alloy impermeable per NFPA chemicals and CW. Protection is provided by barrier material.

Stock Number — 82330

Protection Type — Percutaneous

Equipment Category — Boots

Availability — Commercially available

Current User(s) — NFPA

Manufacturer —
Tingley Rubber Corporation
200 South Avenue
P.O. Box 100
South Plainfield, NJ 07080
800–631–5493 (Tel)
908–631–5498 (Tel)
908–757–9239 (Fax)

Manufacturer Type — Domestic

Developer — Tingley Rubber Corporation

Source — Tingley Rubber Corporation

Certification — Safety Equipment Institute (SEI)

Operational Parameters

Chemical Warfare (CW) Agents Protected Against — Nerve—GA, GB, GD, GF, and VX; blister—H, HD, HN, L

Biological Warfare (BW) Agents Protected Against — Classical BW agents: Anthrax, typhus, ricin, and ebola

Toxic Industrial (TIMs) Protected Against — TIMs protected: 21 chemical family groups

Duration of Protection — CW protection—6 h. TIMs—1 h minimum in each of the 21 chemical groups.

Recommended Use(s) — Tactical operations and crisis management

Physical Parameters

Sizes Available — Sizes 7 through 13

Weight — 6.66 lb

Package Size and Volume — 12.5 in x 18.5 in x 5.5 in

Power Requirements — Not applicable

Material Type	Fire retardant PVC alloy impermeable per NFPA chemicals and CW
Construction Type	Seamless construction
Color	Orange upper with yellow sole
Logistical Parameters	
Ease of Use	Highly mobile, flexible, and compatible with encapsulated suits
Consumables	Not applicable
Maintenance Requirements	Check for cuts and damage after use
Shelf Life	Shelf life indefinite. Critical temperature over 250 °F for extended time.
Transportability	Transportable and compatible with life support equipment
Operational Limitations	No detrimental effect for extended service at temperature of 50 °F, 70 °F, and 90 °F
Environmental Conditions	Designed to be worn in common outdoor weather conditions and climates
Unit Cost	$56
Maintenance Cost	Observation of any significant damage
Warranty	Tingley warrants the boot to be free of defects in material and workmanship for 3 yr. This warrantee does not cover industrial and commercial use or damage thereof.
Don/Doff Information	No assistance required in don/doff
Use/Reuse	May be reused if not contaminated or damaged. Rinse off with mud, soap, and water.
Launderability	Depending on chemical contamination, may be rinsed and reused several times
Accessories	Not applicable
Special Requirements	
Training Requirements	Don/doff precycle
Training Available	Not required, other than damage assessment upon use
Manuals Available	Hang tag on each pair
Surveillance Testing Requirements	Inspection for cuts, damage, and chemical contamination
Support Equipment	Not applicable
Testing Information	Tested chemical and physically per NFPA/SEI available
Applicable Regulations	Not applicable
Health Hazards	Not applicable
Communications Interface Capability	Compatible with fully encapsulated suits
EOD Compatibility	Compatible with EOD suits in a CB environment

General

Name — *Weapons of Mass Destruction (WMD) Contamination Containment Bag*

Item # 69

Picture Not Available

Technology	Impermeable, specialty laminate. Contains thermoplastic materials. Is self-extinguishing. Protection is provided by barrier material.
Stock Number	None
Protection Type	Percutaneous
Equipment Category	Miscellaneous
Availability	Commercially available. In production since 1980.
Current User(s)	Office of Special Technology, field trials ongoing
Manufacturer	ILC Dover, Inc. One Moonwalker Rd. Frederica, DE 19946–2080 POC: Rhonda Haller 800–931–9567 (Tel)
Manufacturer Type	Domestic
Developer	ILC Dover, Inc.
Source	ILC Dover, Inc.
Certification	Not applicable

Operational Parameters

Chemical Warfare (CW) Agents Protected Against	Effective against all standard military agents such as G agents, VX, HD, and CK
Biological Warfare (BW) Agents Protected Against	Protection levels tested to a PF of >10000, which renders the system effective against biological agents. The material used for the overpack bags is also used in a level A suit in operation by the CDC.
Toxic Industrial (TIMs) Protected Against	Performance to be determined, but material used is inherently resistant to chemical permeation and damage induced by exposure to toxic chemicals (this material is used in a Level A suit, suitable for industrial chemical use)
Duration of Protection	>3 h
Recommended Use(s)	Not specified

Physical Parameters

Sizes Available	3 sizes: small: 11 in x 42 in, medium: 22 in x 94 in, and large: 44 in x 144 in
Weight	Maximum < 2 lb
Package Size and Volume	Maximum size of packaged overpack bag is 44 in x ~3 in x ~3 in, depending on size selected
Power Requirements	Not applicable
Material Type	Impermeable, specialty laminate. Contains thermoplastic materials. Is self-extinguishing. The laminate material is designed specifically to be highly resistant to puncture and rough handling.
Construction Type	Heat sealed seam construction

Color	Light blue
Logistical Parameters	
Ease of Use	Bags can be sealed easily while wearing MOPP4 gear, specifically gloves
Consumables	None
Maintenance Requirements	None
Shelf Life	5 yr to 10 yr
Transportability	Transportable via air, ground, or sea
Operational Limitations	Operational environment: 32 °F to 125 °F Storage environment: -20 °F to 165 °F Resistant and operable in salt fog, high/low humidity, and rain environments
Environmental Conditions	Laminate material will give off toxic vapors during combustion
Unit Cost	Small: $150/ea Medium: $250/ea Large: $540/ea
Maintenance Cost	None
Warranty	90 d on defects in materials and workmanship
Don/Doff Information	Not applicable
Use/Reuse	Disposable after one exposure
Launderability	Article is not launderable, but can be decontaminated to prevent contamination of the user during operation
Accessories	None
Special Requirements	
Training Requirements	Very low
Training Available	As required
Manuals Available	None
Surveillance Testing Requirements	No maintenance is required
Support Equipment	None
Testing Information	Test data was generated during the WMD contract through the USA Material Command and Acquisition Center, contract # DAAD05-98-C-0023
Applicable Regulations	Not applicable
Health Hazards	Not applicable
Communications Interface Capability	Not specified
EOD Compatibility	Not specified

General

Name — *Chemical-Biological Eye/Respiratory Disposable (C-BERD) Hood/Mask*

Item # 70

Picture Not Available

Technology — Impermeable, specialty laminate. Is partially flammable, but self-extinguishes itself.

Stock Number — None

Protection Type — Percutaneous/respiratory

Equipment Category — Hood/mask

Availability — Commercially available; 600 units of military configuration delivered to SO/LIC. Commercial version in low to medium quantities available in 3 mo to 6 mo, pending on order.

Current User(s) — SO/LIC, Saudi Arabia

Manufacturer — ILC Dover, Inc.
One Moonwalker Rd.
Frederica, DE 19946–2080
POC: Rhonda Haller
800–931–9567 (Tel)

Manufacturer Type — Domestic

Developer — ILC Dover, Inc.

Source — ILC Dover, Inc.

Certification — We intend to submit the C-BERD, along with past test data, to SBCCOM in April for testing under their Test Support Agreement (TSA) program. Upon completion of the TSA, we will submit C-BERD for NIOSH certification.

Operational Parameters

Chemical Warfare (CW) Agents Protected Against — Protection against GB, GD, VX, HD, CK, and riot control agents such as CS

Biological Warfare (BW) Agents Protected Against — >99.99 % filtration efficiency against biological agents, simulated using polydispersed corn oil aerosol with MMAD of 0.4 μ to 0.6 μ

Toxic Industrial (TIMs) Protected Against — Protection against TIMs can be tailored by the addition of filter snap-ons. This capability warrants further discussion.

Duration of Protection — > 2 h

Recommended Use(s) — Not specified

Physical Parameters

Sizes Available — 1 size fits all

Weight — 1.2 lb as worn

Package Size and Volume — < 12 in x 5 in x 1.5 in packaged size possible with vacuum packing

Power Requirements — Not applicable

Material Type — Impermeable, specialty laminate. Is partially flammable, but self-extinguishes itself. In packaged state, resistant to rough handling as simulated by Q113 tumbler. As worn, mask is resistant to typical military rough handling and operation.

Construction Type	Heat sealed seam construction
Color	Semi-transparent
Logistical Parameters	
Ease of Use	Mask does not restrict FOV, range of motion, or introduce excessive wearer encumbrance. > 2 h of wear are tolerable from a comfort standpoint.
Consumables	None
Maintenance Requirements	None
Shelf Life	5 yr to 10 yr
Transportability	Transportable via air, ground, or sea
Operational Limitations	Operational temperature: -20 °F to 125 °F. Storage temperature: -65 °F to 165 °F. Resistant and operable in salt fog, high/low humidity, and rain environments.
Environmental Conditions	Mask material will give off toxic vapors during combustion
Unit Cost	$50 to $75 per unit, in high volume
Maintenance Cost	None
Warranty	90 d on defects in materials and workmanship
Don/Doff Information	No assistance needed; self-donning and doffing within 15 sec
Use/Reuse	Disposable after one exposure
Launderability	Article is not launderable. Mask can be decontaminated to allow for CCA doffing.
Accessories	None
Special Requirements	
Training Requirements	Very low—follow donning directions on label
Training Available	As required
Manuals Available	Training/operations manual is available
Surveillance Testing Requirements	No maintenance is required
Support Equipment	None
Testing Information	Test data generated during a formal qualification effort for the Air Force on the DERP program, Contract # F33657–92–C–2116. See attached additional data pertaining to requirements of the product and actual data obtained.
Applicable Regulations	Not applicable
Health Hazards	No skin toxicity or similar issues have been identified
Communications Interface Capability	Not specified
EOD Compatibility	Not specified

General

Name	*ILC Model 15 Cool Vest*
Item # 71	
Technology	Permeable, flame retardant cotton or Nomex. Cool Vest Nomex material is a highly flame retardant fabric.
Stock Number	Model 15
Protection Type	Personal cooling
Equipment Category	Ice pack vest is a lightweight, low-profile static cooling garment. It is fully insulated self-contained garment that uses frozen gel packs to help prevent heat stress, keeping workers cool in high ambient temperatures. Can be used in explosive Class I and Class II environments.
Availability	Commercially available. In production since 1990.
Current User(s)	EAI Inc. 1308 Continental Drive, Ste. J Abingdon, MD 21009
Manufacturer	ILC Dover, Inc. One Moonwalker Rd. Frederica, DE 19946–2080 POC: Rhonda Haller 800–931–9567 (Tel)
Manufacturer Type	Domestic
Developer	ILC Dover, Inc.
Source	ILC Dover, Inc. Haller@ilcdover.com
Certification	Not applicable

Operational Parameters

Chemical Warfare (CW) Agents Protected Against	None
Biological Warfare (BW) Agents Protected Against	None
Toxic Industrial (TIMs) Protected Against	None
Duration of Protection	4 h to 6 h
Recommended Use(s)	Suggested applications: Under protective clothing, nuclear plants, agricultural workers, gas utilities, medical maladies, and sports mascots.

Physical Parameters

Sizes Available	1 size fits all
Weight	8 lb
Package Size and Volume	21 in x 12 in x 12 in
Power Requirements	Not applicable
Material Type	Permeable, flame retardant cotton or Nomex. Cool Vest Nomex material is a highly flame retardant fabric. Extremely durable.
Construction Type	Sewn seams
Color	Light blue

Logistical Parameters

Ease of Use	Wearing: The Ice Pack Vest is secured in the front via velcro straps. Six strips of frozen gel packs are inserted into the 6 horizontal pockets (3 front, 3 back) in the vest. Velcro seam on the left shoulder makes it easy to put on.
Consumables	None
Maintenance Requirements	None
Shelf Life	>10 yr
Transportability	Transportable via air, ground, or sea
Operational Limitations	Not applicable
Environmental Conditions	Not specified
Unit Cost	$209
Maintenance Cost	$0
Warranty	90 d on defects in materials and workmanship
Don/Doff Information	Features: Self-contained, durable, insulated vest, low profile, weighs 5 lb to 8 lb fully loaded, takes seconds to put-on/remove, split shoulder design.
Use/Reuse	Unlimited reuse
Launderability	Machine launderable with mild soap. Air dry.
Accessories	Replacement gel strips (5 oz or 9 oz)

Special Requirements

Training Requirements	None
Training Available	None required
Manuals Available	User's manual included with each unit
Surveillance Testing Requirements	None required
Support Equipment	Freezer
Testing Information	Available upon request
Applicable Regulations	Not applicable
Health Hazards	None
Communications Interface Capability	Not specified
EOD Compatibility	Not specified

General

Name — *ILC Model 19 Cool Vest*

Item # 72

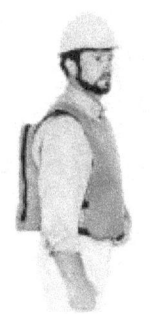

Technology — Through the use of a centrifugal pump, chilled water is circulated throughout the series of passages within the vest. All mechanical components are packaged within the vest to provide an effective, compact system.

Stock Number — Model 19

Protection Type — Personal cooling

Equipment Category — The ILC Model 19 Cool Vest is a completely portable cooling garment worn to aid in maintaining worker comfort and safety in extremely warm environments for extended periods of time. External bypass valve control water temperature for continuous water circulation.

Availability — Commercially available. In production since 1990.

Current User(s) — EAI Inc.
1308 Continental Drive, Ste. J
Abingdon, MD 21009

Manufacturer — ILC Dover, Inc.
One Moonwalker Rd.
Frederica, DE 19946–2080
POC: Rhonda Haller
800–931–9567 (Tel)

Manufacturer Type — Domestic

Developer — ILC Dover, Inc.

Source — ILC Dover, Inc.
Haller@ilcdover.com

Certification — Not applicable

Operational Parameters

Chemical Warfare (CW) Agents Protected Against — None

Biological Warfare (BW) Agents Protected Against — None

Toxic Industrial (TIMs) Protected Against — None

Duration of Protection — The cooling bag stores water, cubed or crushed ice, or reusable ice packs giving an average of 1 h of cooling during normal work cycles. An 8 V rechargeable battery gives up to 3 h of continuous operation. Battery charger and additional battery packs are available.

Recommended Use(s) — Foundries, forgeries, and theme park characters

Physical Parameters

Sizes Available	1 size fits all
Weight	Weighs 10 lb fully loaded
Package Size and Volume	Not specified
Power Requirements	8 V rechargeable battery gives up to 3 h of continuous operation. Battery charger and additional battery packs are available.
Material Type	Blue urethane coated nylon shell
Construction Type	Sewn seams
Color	Light blue

Logistical Parameters

Ease of Use	The pocket housing the pump, ice bag, and battery pack can be worn on the back or front, enabling the user to wear it alone, with a breathing system, or under a protective clothing ensemble
Consumables	8 V rechargeable battery
Maintenance Requirements	None
Shelf Life	>10 yr
Transportability	Transportable via air, ground, or sea
Operational Limitations	The ILC Model 19 Cool Vest is a completely portable cooling garment worn to aid in maintaining worker comfort and safety in extremely warm environments for extended periods of time
Environmental Conditions	Not specified
Unit Cost	$284
Maintenance Cost	$0
Warranty	90 d on defects in materials and workmanship
Don/Doff Information	The pocket housing the pump, ice bag, and battery pack can be worn on the back or front, enabling the user to wear it alone, with a breathing system, or under a protective clothing ensemble
Use/Reuse	Unlimited reuse
Launderability	Mechanical components can be removed, allowing the vest to be machine laundered
Accessories	Battery charger, reusable ice pack, and battery

Special Requirements

Training Requirements	None
Training Available	None required
Manuals Available	User's manual included with each unit
Surveillance Testing Requirements	None required
Support Equipment	Freezer
Testing Information	Available upon request
Applicable Regulations	Not applicable
Health Hazards	None
Communications Interface Capability	Not specified
EOD Compatibility	Not specified

General

Name *Personal Ice Cooling System (PICS)*

Item # 73

Technology	Liquid cooling shirt is cotton/polyester blend with PVC tubing. Shirt is permeable however it is not designed to be a primary protective layer.
Stock Number	PICS: 8415–01–455–3175 PICS Shirt (SM): 8415–01–465–3766 PICS Shirt (M): 8415–-01–465–3767 PICS Shirt (L): 8415–01–465–0121 PICS Shirt (XL): 8415–01–465–0120
Protection Type	Heat stress management
Equipment Category	Cooling system
Availability	Fielding in process (December 1999 through July 2002). Army EOD units, technical escort units and chemical storage sites will be fielded equipment.
Current User(s)	EOD units, Technical Escort Units, and chemical activities
Manufacturer	GEOMET Technologies, Inc. 20251 Century Blvd. Germantown, MD 20874 301–428–9898 (Tel) POC: Jef Harris
Manufacturer Type	Domestic
Developer	GEOMET Technologies, Inc., Germantown, MD, and Natick Research Development and Engineering Center (NRDEC), Kansas Street, Natick, MA
Source	GEOMET Technologies, Inc.
Certification	Type Classified by the U.S. Army, 1997

Operational Parameters

Chemical Warfare (CW) Agents Protected Against	The PICS is designed to be worn with chemical protective clothing such as the STEPO and ITAP chemical protective suits. External components of the PICS have been tested to protect against GB and HD.
Biological Warfare (BW) Agents Protected Against	No testing was conducted against BW agents. However, the PICS was designed to operate in a CW environment, therefore it is a safe assumption that the PICS (when worn with appropriate protective clothing such as the STEPO or ITAP chemical protective suits.
Toxic Industrial (TIMs) Protected Against	None tested
Duration of Protection	4 h mission duration

Recommended Use(s)	For use in chemical environments with encapsulating suits and other protective clothing where heat stress is a concern
Physical Parameters	
Sizes Available	Liquid cooling shirts available in 4 sizes: S, M, L, and XL
Weight	13 lb (mission ready)
Package Size and Volume	12 in x 12 in x 18 in
Power Requirements	3 D cell batteries. 4 h to 6 h operation between battery change-out. Ice bottles must be frozen solid prior to use for optimal cooling.
Material Type	Liquid cooling shirt is cotton/polyester blend with PVC tubing. Shirt is permeable however it is not designed to be a primary protective layer. The PICS should be worn with protective clothing when contact with hazardous chemicals or CW agents is expected.
Construction Type	Not applicable
Color	OD green pump and white ice bag (external components)
Logistical Parameters	
Ease of Use	Compatible with STEPO and ITAP chemical protective suits. Simple to use and maintain.
Consumables	3 D cell batteries. Water must be frozen in the system ice bottles before use. Water is also circulated through the PICS during operation. The water can be reused, however, it must be refrozen in the ice bottles.
Maintenance Requirements	Laundering of liquid cooling shirt, freezing of ice bottles, visual inspection, and leak test
Shelf Life	None determined. Manufacturer recommends inspecting rubber parts closely after 5 yr.
Transportability	Soft carry bag. Also ice bag tote bag available to transport ice refills at work site.
Operational Limitations	The PICS is used in elevated temperatures to manage heat stress and reduce the increase of the user's core temperature. There is no operating temperature range specified for PICS. Moderately durable.
Environmental Conditions	None
Unit Cost	PICS: 1 to 100, $2.2K; 101 to 250, $2.1K; 251 to 500, and $2K PICS Service Kit: $207 Ice Bag Tote Bag: $56
Maintenance Cost	1 man h/use and 4 man h/yr for quarterly inspections (based on information in TM 10–8415–232–23&P Maintenance Allocation Chart)
Warranty	1 yr with the exception of liquid cooling shirt. Liquid cooling shirt is warranted for 3 mo.
Don/Doff Information	Requires one assistant when donning/doffing with chemical protective clothing
Use/Reuse	Reusable
Launderability	Decon in accordance with DA PAM 385–61 and AR 385–61. Do not use DS2 or sodium hydroxide for decontamination. Ice bag, ice bottle and external coolant tether must be decontaminated for disposal if exposed to CW agent vapor or liquid contamination. Pump unit may be decontaminated if exposed to CW agent vapor contamination. If pump unit is exposed to CW agent liquid contamination pump must be decontaminated for disposal. Launder shirt using nonphosphate soap, warm water, and air dry.

Accessories	3 ice bottles, 3 ice bags, and 3 coupling caps

Special Requirements

Training Requirements	Minimum of 4 hr for operation. Additional 8 h for maintenance.
Training Available	Yes
Manuals Available	Technical manual TM 10-8415-232-23&P developed under Government contract to support operation and maintenance
Surveillance Testing Requirements	Visual inspection, vacuum test, and operational checks IAW TM 3-4240-351-23&P. All materials to conduct tests are included in PICS Service Kit.
Support Equipment	Liquid coolant passthrough is required when used with encapsulating suits such as the STEPO and ITAP chemical protective suits
Testing Information	CW agent data available from NRDEC. (Refer to coolant pass through in component testing information for PICS data).
Applicable Regulations	Safety precautions are identified in TM 10-8415-232-23&P
Health Hazards	None
Communications Interface Capability	Not applicable
EOD Compatibility	Yes. Specifically designed for use with STEPO and ITAP systems. Also compatible with other protective clothing.

General

Name *Flexi ICE Cold Vest*

Item # 74

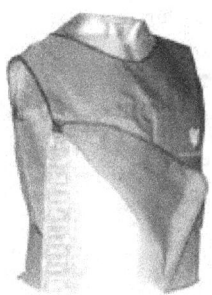

Technology — Flexi ICE Cold Vest is a cooling system incorporating four cooling elements inserted within a lightweight vest. It is worn under the tunic and over the underwear. An outer Nomex fabric and an inner cotton fabric make it both comfortable and resistant to heat and flames.

Stock Number — Big Flexi Ice package 98 075–01 includes: 8 Flexi Ice Cold Vests, 1 freezer box, and 2 cool bags. Small Flexi Ice package 98 076–01 includes: 4 Flexi Ice Cold Vest and 1 cool bag.

Protection Type — Heat stress management

Equipment Category — Cooling system

Availability — Fielding in process (December 1999 through July 2002). Army EOD units, technical escort units and chemical storage sites will be fielded equipment.

Current User(s) — Swedish Rescue Service Agency (SRSA)

Manufacturer — INTERSPIRO INC.
31 Business Park Drive
Branford, CT 06405
800–468–7788 or 203–481–3899 (Tel)
203–483–1879 (Fax)

Manufacturer Type — International

Developer — Interspiro

Source — http://www.interspiro.com

Certification — Not specified

Operational Parameters

Chemical Warfare (CW) Agents Protected Against — Not specified

Biological Warfare (BW) Agents Protected Against — Not specified

Toxic Industrial (TIMs) Protected Against — None tested.

Duration of Protection — Action time 30 min to 2 h. Deep freezing from 60 s with freezer box.

Recommended Use(s) — When working in extreme conditions

Physical Parameters

Sizes Available	S and L
Weight	Lightweight—less than 2.2 lb
Package Size and Volume	Not specified
Power Requirements	Not specified
Material Type	An outer Nomex fabric and an inner cotton fabric make it both comfortable and resistant to heat and flames
Construction Type	Not applicable
Color	Blue

Logistical Parameters

Ease of Use	The cooling elements can be quickly frozen within our specially developed freezer box. With the freezer box connected to a standard CO_2 fire extinguisher, the cooling elements freeze within approximately 60 s, giving up to 1 h of use. It is of course also possible to freeze the cooling elements in a standard deep freeze.
Consumables	Standard CO2 fire extinguisher
Maintenance Requirements	Not specified
Shelf Life	Not specified
Transportability	For transportation and storage, for up to 12 h, the system includes a Cool Bag. The Cool Bag is designed for four Flexi Ice Cold Vests.
Operational Limitations	Fire fighters pulse rates decreased and body temperature and perspiration reduced
Environmental Conditions	None
Unit Cost	Not specified
Maintenance Cost	Not specified
Warranty	Not specified
Don/Doff Information	Not specified
Use/Reuse	Quick to recharge and reuse. With the freezer box connected to a standard CO_2 fire extinguisher, the cooling elements freeze within approximately 60 s, giving up to 1 h of use.
Launderability	The vest is washable—even with the cooling elements inserted
Accessories	Cool bag, freezer box, and cool bags

Special Requirements

Training Requirements	Not specified
Training Available	Yes
Manuals Available	Not specified
Surveillance Testing Requirements	Not specified
Support Equipment	Standard freezer
Testing Information	Vigorous tests conducted by the Swedish National Institute of Working Life, at the request of the Swedish Rescue Service Agency (SRSA)
Applicable Regulations	Not specified
Health Hazards	None
Communications Interface Capability	Not applicable
EOD Compatibility	Not specified, but can be used with fire fighting equipment

ABOUT THE LAW ENFORCEMENT AND CORRECTIONS STANDARDS AND TESTING PROGRAM

The Law Enforcement and Corrections Standards and Testing Program is sponsored by the Office of Science and Technology of the National Institute of Justice (NIJ), U.S. Department of Justice. The program responds to the mandate of the Justice System Improvement Act of 1979, directed NIJ to encourage research and development to improve the criminal justice system and to disseminate the results to Federal, State, and local agencies.

The Law Enforcement and Corrections Standards and Testing Program is an applied research effort that determines the technological needs of justice system agencies, sets minimum performance standards for specific devices, tests commercially available equipment against those standards, and disseminates the standards and the test results to criminal justice agencies nationally and internationally.

The program operates through:

The *Law Enforcement and Corrections Technology Advisory Council* (LECTAC), consisting of nationally recognized criminal justice practitioners from Federal, State, and local agencies, which assesses technological needs and sets priorities for research programs and items to be evaluated and tested.

The *Office of Law Enforcement Standards* (OLES) at the National Institute of Standards and Technology, which develops voluntary national performance standards for compliance testing to ensure that individual items of equipment are suitable for use by criminal justice agencies. The standards are based upon laboratory testing and evaluation of representative samples of each item of equipment to determine the key attributes, develop test methods, and establish minimum performance requirements for each essential attribute. In addition to the highly technical standards, OLES also produces technical reports and user guidelines that explain in nontechnical terms the capabilities of available equipment.

The *National Law Enforcement and Corrections Technology Center* (NLECTC), operated by a grantee, which supervises a national compliance testing program conducted by independent laboratories. The standards developed by OLES serve as performance benchmarks against which commercial equipment is measured. The facilities, personnel, and testing capabilities of the independent laboratories are evaluated by OLES prior to testing each item of equipment, and OLES helps the NLECTC staff review and analyze data. Test results are published in Equipment Performance Reports designed to help justice system procurement officials make informed purchasing decisions.

Publications are available at no charge through the National Law Enforcement and Corrections Technology Center. Some documents are also available online through the Internet/World Wide Web. To request a document or additional information, call 800–248–2742 or 301–519–5060, or write:

> National Law Enforcement and Corrections Technology Center
> P.O. Box 1160
> Rockville, MD 20849–1160
> E-Mail: *asknlectc@nlectc.org*
> World Wide Web address: *http://www.nlectc.org*

This document is not intended to create, does not create, and may not be relied upon to create any rights, substantive or procedural, enforceable at law by any party in any matter civil or criminal.

Opinions or points of view expressed in this document represent a consensus of the authors and do not represent the official position or policies of the U.S. Department of Justice. The products and manufacturers discussed in this document are presented for informational purposes only and do not constitute product approval or endorsement by the U.S. Department of Justice.

The National Institute of Justice is a component of the Office of Justice Programs, which also includes the Bureau of Justice Assistance, the Bureau of Justice Statistics, the Office of Juvenile Justice and Delinquency Prevention, and the Office for Victims of Crime.